THE
ALEXANDER
TECHNIQUE

THE
ALEXANDER
TECHNIQUE

Liz Hodgkinson

PIATKUS

© Liz Hodgkinson 1988

First published in 1988 by
Judy Piatkus (Publishers) Ltd,
5 Windmill Street, London W1P 1HF

Reprinted 1989
Reprinted 1990

British Library Cataloguing in Publication Data

Hodgkinson, Liz
  The Alexander technique.
  1. Physical fitness. Posture. Theories of
  Alexander F. Matthias
  I. Title
  613.7′8′0924

  ISBN 0-86188-709-3
  ISBN 0-86188-807-3 (Pbk)

Designed by Sue Ryall
Illustrated by Linda Broad

Phototypeset in 11/12pt Linotron Baskerville by
Phoenix Photosetting, Chatham
Printed and bound in Great Britain by
Mackays of Chatham PLC, Chatham, Kent

Contents

Dedication

This book is gratefully dedicated to Lilian Carpenter

Introduction

Over the past few years the Alexander Technique has become one of the most popular alternative therapies, with specialised clinics and treatment rooms being set up all over the country. But, you may ask, what exactly is the treatment? How does it work? And why has it become so very popular?

I'll answer the last question first, because it is the easiest. The Technique is popular quite simply because it works – and it has stood the test of time. It was formulated almost 100 years ago by an Australian actor named Frederick Matthias Alexander.

The Alexander Technique is basically a series of physical movements designed to correct bad posture and bring the body back into alignment, thus helping it to function efficiently, as nature intended. The Technique can be used to alleviate a variety of mental, emotional and physical conditions. Most often it is used for complaints which ordinary medical treatment cannot seem to help. People may consult an Alexander teacher if they suffer from bad backache, rheumatism, arthritis, asthma, or depression – and have already tried treatments suggested by their doctor. The idea is that, once you have learned to move your muscles and joints correctly, various ills of the body caused by wrong movement can then start to right themselves. The Technique is necessary, and has become popular, because the vast majority of us move our bodies wrongly – often without realising that we are doing so, until health problems arise.

Consequence of bad habits

Although the Alexander Technique is primarily a physical therapy, it has little to do with simple keep-fit or relaxation. Rather, it consists of unlearning bad habits which may have been acquired over many years of daily use, and have therefore become almost second nature. It seeks to replace wrong postures and muscular use with correct usage. A trained Alexander teacher will instruct pupils in this correct usage.

Alexander himself believed that most of humanity's ills – mental, emotional and physical – are caused by the gradual and largely unconscious acquisition of bad habits. When we are very small children, he said, we stand, move and conduct ourselves correctly. But all children learn by imitation, copying the behaviour of the adults around them. In consequence they learn to move wrongly, to sit wrongly and to conduct themselves wrongly. The vast majority of adults, Alexander believed, conduct themselves physically in ways which are far from ideal, and predispose the body to illness and malfunctions of various kinds. Most adults, he stated, have terrible posture, and put the wrong kind of effort into every physical action.

Alexander teachers estimate that by adolescence, about 90 per cent of us have got into bad habits of walking, sitting and standing that have become so ingrained they feel natural – and most of us cannot imagine any other way of doing things.

Unfortunately, the longer a bad habit persists, the more difficult it becomes to break, and the danger is that as we gradually acquire wrong ways of walking, sitting or even speaking, our bodies will become deformed. For many years, this deformity may not be noticed, then suddenly, there will be a twinge, or perhaps an agonising backache. Only then may we realise that something is wrong. The kind of deformity which comes gradually is usually very apparent by old age, but the bent posture and crooked backs of many elderly people are *not* inevitable consequences of growing old – just warnings of what can happen, if we do not take care.

By the stage that bad backache has become a problem, there is not much point in going to the doctor for pills. Although these may alleviate the pain, they do not constitute a cure. The problem will continue to get worse because pills cannot undo the bad habits of a lifetime. The only way to get better, say Alexander teachers, is to unlearn the bad habit, by substituting a good one.

How the Technique works

An Alexander teacher will ask her pupil to perform certain ordinary, everyday actions, such as sitting, standing, and walking across the room. As the pupil sits, stands and walks, the teacher will observe closely what is happening. She will then instruct the pupil how to sit down, to stand, and to walk in the correct way – the way in which the body was designed by nature to behave.

At first, the pupil may not be able to do as the teacher instructs. Bad postural habits can set in very early in life, even at the age of five or six. So by the time a 40-year-old adult with excruciating backache comes for Alexander lessons, there may be 35 years of wrong posture to correct.

The Alexander Technique can only start to work when a pupil begins to 'feel the difference'. With practice, the correct posture can be attained, and maintained, and good habits start to take the place of the bad ones. Then the chronic health problem can begin to clear up.

Although the Technique is primarily physical, it can also help all kinds of mental conditions. Alexander believed that all humans hold emotional states within their bodies. Therefore, if you can correct the physical imbalance, he reasoned, you also stand a chance of correcting the mental state which is causing unhappiness or anxiety. In this way, the Alexander Technique constitutes the complete opposite approach from, say, psychoanalysis, or Freudian therapy.

Instead of working on the mind, the Alexander teacher works on the body. The idea behind this is that it is basically fear, anxiety, tension and stress which make people adopt wrong postures in the first place. For example, somebody who is nervous and afraid, or lacking in self-confidence may walk around slightly stooped or with the head hunched in their shoulders, as if to hide themselves. Even quite small children may do this. Or, a person who is very angry may put far more effort into every action than is really needed. In time, chronic anger will have a physical effect, so that overdoing actions will become normal, and natural.

Alexander believed that many human characteristics are simply learned habits, rather than innate aspects; and every time we perform an everyday action wrongly, we deepen the habit still further. One example of this is stammering, an affliction which is notoriously difficult to cure. People stammer, said Alexander, *not* because there is anything wrong with their vocal cords, but because they have got into the habit of stammering. As people use speech all the time, it is difficult to break the stammering habit, once it has set in.

The more often we have to perform any action, the more difficult it becomes to correct. We can see this easily in every-day life. Every day, we all perform actions that are repeated so often we never even think about them. Just reflect for a minute on how you sit. Do you just plonk yourself into a chair? Do you automatically cross your legs? Do you do anything special with your hands? The chances are, you just don't know.

How do you clean your teeth? Do you pick up the tooth-paste first, or the toothbrush? Do you brush the top or the bottom teeth first? How long do you take over the task? Again, you probably don't know. You clean your teeth so often that the process has become automatic. It is likely that you never give much thought, either, to how you wash your hands, or hold the telephone.

What happens, though, is that all these everyday, uncon-sidered actions can in time set up serious imbalances in the body. We are simply not aware of these because they have come to feel right. We can, argued Alexander, acquire any kind of habit, good or bad. Anything at all can become a habit, if repeated often enough. As the way we walk, stand and sit eventually become habits, so do our mental and emotional reactions. We can get into the habit of reacting with anger to everything, of being bad-tempered, of scowling rather than smiling. We can get into the habit of feeling sorry for our-selves, believing that nothing is ever going to go right – or by contrast, we can acquire the habit of positive thinking.

Above all, the Alexander Technique teaches people to replace bad, negative habits with good, positive ones so that they will be able to achieve their full potential, mentally, physically and emotionally. One key to the Alexander Technique is understanding that you cannot separate mind and body; they are inextricably bound up with each other.

Importance of the spine

It all starts with the spine, rather than in the head. The Technique teaches that if we learn to use our spines correctly, then we will be able to rid ourselves of both physical and mental ills. This is because every organ in the body, including the brain, is directly or indirectly attached to the spine, which Alexander called the area of 'primary control'.

What goes on in the spine largely determines both mental and physical health. Just try this simple test. Sit comfortably in a chair. Now slump forward and put your hands to your head in an attitude of dejection. Notice how you immediately feel miserable and depressed?

Now sit upright and lengthen your spine by imagining that a string is coming out of the top of your head and pulling you towards the ceiling. As you do this, smile. You will notice that, instantly, your mood lifts and you feel happier. The reason for this is that inside you, many complicated but beneficial biochemical and physical changes are taking place.

Humans are not meant to be slumped and dejected, but upright, healthy and happy. However, in order to become supremely healthy, it is essential to be aware of our bodies, and what they are trying to tell us.

To sum up, the basic principles of the Alexander Technique are:

- To regain or maintain health, we must be completely aware of our bodies and how they function; otherwise, we cannot make changes to improve our condition. The Alexander Technique teaches a new awareness of our body which may have been lost by years of bad habits.

- Muscle action is not simple reflex; muscles move in response to mental action. The second you start to think about moving a muscle, it begins to move. The Alexander

Technique teaches you how to instruct your muscles to move correctly, to become aware of what they are doing and how they work.

- Because bad postural habits are often acquired early in childhood and repeated endlessly, we may be hurting ourselves and putting our bodies out of alignment without realising it. Eventually, though, our bodies will complain and let us know they are being mistreated. Alexander teachers will help you to correct bad posture.

- The parts of the body do not all act independently of each other. Inevitably, whatever happens to one part will in time affect other areas. For instance, if you put an inappropriate amount of effort into cleaning your teeth three times a day, eventually you may be seized up with backache – a condition seemingly unrelated to a simple matter of daily hygiene.

- Habits are not reflexes; they have been learned until they become automatic. But as a habit can be learned, so it can be unlearned. The best way of unlearning a bad habit is to replace it by a good one, and practise the good habit until that becomes innate in its turn.

- Most people imagine they have no control over their habits. In fact, they can always be changed – no matter how long they have been part of your life.

- The Alexander Technique believes that the process is more important than the end result. For example: the way you sit down is more important than actually achieving the position of sitting. Above all, the technique teaches people to become consciously aware of the ways in which they do everyday tasks. For an Alexander teacher, there is no such thing as an unimportant physical task – everything matters. You learn to replace unconscious habits by conscious control, and in doing so, pave the way for optimum health and maximum achievement of potential.

Find a reputable teacher

Over the years, the Alexander Technique has acquired a reputation for being difficult to understand, describe and do. In fact, it is very easy to understand – once you have grasped the basic principles. However, like anything else in life worth doing, it takes practice.

There's no doubt that it is worth the effort. Although the Technique is not a wonder cure for all ills, anybody can benefit to some degree from an understanding of the principles. All of us acquire bad habits over the years which we would be far better off without.

It has to be understood, though, that the Alexander Technique is not primarily a self-help therapy. Those who suffer from a specific complaint should go to a reputable teacher for lessons. The rest of us can learn better and more efficient ways of undertaking everyday tasks – and how to prevent the deformities and disabilities that can otherwise occur in later life.

There is no age, sex or disability limit. Anybody can benefit from an understanding of the technique. You have nothing to lose but your own bad habits!

1

The Technique
and the man

To appreciate the Alexander Technique fully, it is essential to know something about the man who formulated it. Frederick Matthias Alexander was born in 1869 in Wynyard, Tasmania, Australia, into a farming family. He was the eldest of eight children, and the family was constantly short of money. Usually called FM, Alexander was apparently a difficult and recalcitrant child. Also, he suffered from respiratory problems and had no formal education after the age of nine. Very early in life however, he developed a love for the theatre, and also learned to train and manage horses. The theatre and horses were to become his lifelong interests.

Alexander had ambitions to become a teacher, but family finances would not allow him to train as one. So, at the age of sixteen he had to go to work in a tin mine. Apparently, he worked so conscientiously that within three years he earned enough to go to Melbourne.

There, he started to give Shakespearean recitals, then very popular. Soon, he had regular audiences, and was making enough money from recitals not to have to return to the mine.

Voice problems

His popularity became so great that he decided to make acting his full time career. Then problems set in. Very often, halfway through a recital, his voice would start to go; once he lost it completely.

He consulted doctor after doctor, but none was able to help. He did not seem to be suffering from any physical disability or condition which could be the cause of the voice loss, so they just advised rest, which was hardly conducive to his career. Still aged only nineteen, FM decided to find out for himself what was wrong.

Self-help and discoveries

He fixed up specially positioned mirrors so that he could watch himself declaiming. After a time, he realised that his loss of voice might have something to do with the way he held his head. He observed that when he started to declaim, he had a tendency to pull his head back and downwards. He became convinced that this was the basic reason for his disability. The problem was, how to stop it, as he was completely unaware of the tendency while he was reciting on stage.

He determined to discover just why he pulled his head back when he spoke in public, and eventually concluded that he had simply got into the habit of wrong 'use'. The only way to change the habit was to substitute a better one – not easy when you are unaware of your movements in the first place. By close observation, Alexander realised that the mental tension and lack of co-ordination which affected his vocal chords were connected with the way his head balanced on his neck. He reasoned therefore that it was not possible to separate mind, body and emotions; all worked together, for good or ill. This theory, then revolutionary, became one of the basic tenets of the Alexander philosophy.

Alexander also came to realise that head, neck and body were all interconnected and that whatever he did with one part of his body, inevitably affected other areas. It seemed that mere willpower, or the wish to do things differently, were not enough to change ingrained habits. Because he had mis-used his body for so long, he could not just decide to change his habits – and so get his voice back.

This led him to the discovery that our sense of what felt right about our bodies was unreliable. It was all too easy to get into bad physical and postural habits, and our bodies would not give us the message that something was wrong – until

9

later. He wrote in his most famous book, *The Use of the Self*

Surely if it is possible for feeling to become untrustworthy as a means of direction, it should be possible to make it trustworthy again.

The only way to overcome his disability, he felt, was to dissociate himself from the sense of what felt right, and to learn new habits by conscious effort. He decided that the only way to improve his voice was to learn how to lengthen his stature, and not to throw his head back. This involved lots of practice, until the new way felt as right as the old had once done, and replaced it. And the only way to do this was not to concentrate on the eventual goal, which was giving a recital, but on getting his head, neck and torso into correct alignment. That is, instead of paying attention to the ends, he concentrated on the means.

All these ideas were later to become incorporated into the Alexander Technique but at this time he was simply working on himself. Through constant practice, and by paying more attention to the way he was doing things than the action itself, Alexander managed to change his ingrained habits by conscious control.

Unforeseen benefits

Alexander's voice problems disappeared and with them many other negative characteristics. Formerly, he had had a fearful temper. Now, as his breathing difficulties disappeared, he acquired a more positive, likeable personality, and his fame as an actor grew. His voice was considered to be especially striking.

Eventually, other actors asked him to give them voice lessons and Alexander began to formulate his ideas into a definite technique which could help other people. At first, all of his pupils were those whose voices were important to their careers. By about 1895 he was combining acting and teaching. As his methods seemed to work, doctors started sending certain patients to him, and before long, these ordinary people outnumbered his theatrical students. As they regained proper 'use' of their bodies, these patients found that their health and emotional problems cleared up. It sounded unlikely – but it worked. What made it even more unlikely was that Alexander was not medically qualified, and had hardly any education, yet he had worked his technique out without any help from medical people, psychologists, physical instructors or voice therapists. He was propounding something completely new and little understood by other health professionals of the time – and was achieving remarkable successes.

Teaching full time

Not long after he had established a steady supply of patients, Alexander decided to give up acting and concentrate on teaching full time. He was still only 25 years old, but he was a charismatic character, tall, slim, good-looking, and full of self-confidence – undoubtedly one of the main reasons for his great success.

Soon he moved to Sydney, and became the director of the Sydney Dramatic and Operatic Conservatorium, where his method of teaching was, as he described it, 'one of changing and controlling reactions'. Once you knew how the body worked, and paid conscious attention to how you were using it, you were in a good position to correct any imbalances and wrong habits, he argued.

At the age of 34 he felt he had to go to London, to spread the word even further, and arrived in England on 4 April, 1904. As in Australia, he had no difficulty in attracting pupils, although for a long time the medical profession remained sceptical.

Among his clients were famous actors and actresses of the day, such as Sir Henry Irving, Lily Blayton, Viola Tree and Lily Langtry, and Alexander liked to give expensive lessons to such clients. However, he also taught those who could not afford to pay the full fees.

Everything went well until 1914, when the outbreak of World War One virtually stopped his flow of pupils. Nothing daunted, Alexander departed for America, where he was soon teaching nine hours a day, his energy seemingly inexhaustible.

Developing new concepts

As time went on, Alexander expanded his doctrines and expostulated on the importance of 'means' rather than 'ends'. This basic tenet of the Alexander philosophy states that the main problem today is that we are all 'endgainers'. We are so impatient to achieve our goals that we give hardly any thought to the 'means whereby' we achieve them. Thus when we sit down, all we think of is the sitting down, not how our body changes position in order to sit down. Alexander taught his pupils to concentrate on the 'means whereby', rather than the end result. It was the journey, he said, rather than the arrival, which mattered.

New Yorkers – always on the lookout for something new and exciting – flocked to Alexander's lessons, and he enjoyed ten years of prosperity and lionisation. He even trained his younger brother, Albert Redden, in the technique. Albert became FM's successor in New York.

Publishing his Technique

By 1924, however, Alexander was being accused of cultism, and returned to England. In London, he established a school for children aged three to eight, as he felt that most problems in later life could be traced back to early childhood.

Alexander also started to write books about his Technique. The first, *Man's Supreme Inheritance*, was published in 1910; it set out for the first time his idea that, in order to be well, Man has to exert conscious control over his mind and body.

His second book, *Constructive Conscious Control of the Individual*, first published in 1923, introduced the concepts of 'endgaining' and 'sensory appreciation'. By this, Alexander means understanding what the five senses are trying to tell us. Much of modern life, he felt, blunted the senses and arrested essential feedback to mind and body.

His most famous book, *The Use of the Self*, published in 1932, explains his theories in detail, and introduces those terms which have become famous to students of the Technique: 'Use' and 'Primary Control'. This short work is generally considered to be Alexander's best and most readable.

Far-reaching ideas

Alexander did not confine himself to describing how the body worked, and how certain emotions might affect particular muscular movements. His books contain many ideas on religion, philosophy, anthropology, education, sociology, evolution, medicine, psychology and behaviour. This intellectual approach endeared him to writers such as Aldous Huxley and Bernard Shaw, and the American educationalist John Dewey. Aldous Huxley became one of Alexander's greatest devotees, and even wrote a fictional portrait of him (the character named Miller) in his famous novel, *Eyeless in Gaza*.

Alexander's philosophical bent had its good and bad sides. While it enabled him to be taken seriously by the great thinkers of the day and to attract those at the very top of their profession, the less positive side of all this was that his Technique was also seen as very esoteric – something that only a few extremely clever people could understand. Unfortunately, this has rather persisted and consequently the Technique is still surrounded by a mystique which, really, it need not have.

Alexander's ideas are accessible to all – through the growing number of qualified teachers. His writings however, can be hard to follow. Another problem was that Alexander invented jargon terms which for him have special and specific meanings. But once the jargon is understood, we can see what good sense his ideas make.

The main ideas

Here is a brief outline of Alexander's main ideas:

If we are to stay well and healthy, he argued, we must concentrate above all, on the 'use of the self', being aware always of how we sit, stand, move and generally conduct ourselves physically. Most people perform daily actions unconsciously, unaware that they may be damaging, even deforming themselves. All activities, said Alexander, involve us in complicated sequences of movement – there is no such thing as a simple action.

We must firstly understand the importance of the spine, for this is where the 'primary control' rests. In order to do its job

13

properly, the spine must be lengthened, never shortened. When the spine is continually shortened, undue strain is put on all limbs and organs.

The neck should always be free from muscle tension. Very many people hold a lot of tension in the neck. This then spreads throughout the body.

The head should be allowed to go forward and up, and never back or down. Throwing one's head back, or allowing it to slump on the chest will eventually put the whole body out of alignment.

The torso should be allowed to lengthen and widen out, and the spine should never be arched. Alexander felt that much of physical education in schools (the rigid upright 'Army' stance and rigid concepts of posture which were current in his day) actually deformed the body and unsuited it to healthy functioning in later life. He rejected conventional exercise as a means of using the body properly.

Because most people have acquired bad habits to such an extent that they seem natural, it would be impossible for the average human to correct bad usage alone. For this reason, initially the teacher at an Alexander lesson will 'stand', 'sit' and 'walk' you. Only when you can feel for yourself how different the new instructions are, can you begin to appreciate the improvement. Once you have acquired new sensory experience of these ordinary, everyday acts, the way is paved for greater improvements.

With practice, the new ways of moving the head, neck and torso can become unconscious habits that replace the bad old ways. When we have proper 'primary control' as Alexander termed it, there is greater freedom of action all round. Sight and hearing and speech all improve, and the deeper breathing which results means that far less effort is needed to move limbs and muscles.

Alexander saw his technique as being rather like tidying up an untidy room. If you can change the manner of your use, he said, you will be able to change the conditions throughout your whole body. He wrote:

One of the most remarkable of man's characteristics is his capacity for becoming used to conditions of any kind, whether good or bad, both

*in the self and the environment. Once he has become used to such con-
ditions, they seem to him both right and natural. This capacity is a
boon when it enables him to adapt himself to conditions which are
desirable, but it may prove a great danger when the conditions are
undesirable. When his sensory appreciation is untrustworthy, it is
possible for him to become so familiar to seriously harmful conditions
of misuse of himself that these malconditions will feel right and
comfortable.*

If we think of this doctrine in terms of addictions, it
becomes clear. The human system does not need or initially
welcome cigarettes, alcohol, sugar or mind-altering drugs. If
we start taking these substances, though, in time the body
adapts and not only begins to need them, but actually cries
out for them. If we are not careful, we can become addicted to
them. Unnatural and harmful substances have come to feel
not only right and natural, but actually necessary.

The human body and mind, Alexander argued, are almost
infinitely adaptable, and most of us are not easily able to tell
the difference between what is right and what is wrong. After a
time, whichever we do will come to seem both natural and
normal, and therefore 'right' for us. This happens with both
body usage and mental functioning.

In *The Use of Self* Alexander himself compared the unconscious acquiring of bad habits in general to something such as
smoking. There was no way, he said, ever to 'satisfy' the urge
to smoke. By contrast, 'Each act of smoking is a stimulus to
the smoking of another. Every time a person abstains from
smoking, he breaks a link in the chain.' He continued: 'The
worse these conditions are in a pupil, and the longer they have
been in existence, the more familiar and right they feel to him,
and the harder it is to teach him to overcome them, no matter
how much he may wish to do so.'

Alexander also realised that proper breathing was important, but never formulated a set of breathing exercises as such.
He felt that bad breathing was only a symptom, never the
main cause of disfunction throughout the body. When a
person breathes wrongly – and like anything else, this can
become an ingrained habit – the 'endgaining' principle is
involved, and a vicious circle is developed. An 'endgainer' is

somebody so impatient to achieve an aim that no attention is paid to the way in which the goal is reached.

Alexander wanted to teach a principle whereby the capacity of the chest would be permanently increased, so that serious illnesses linked to chest function could not develop. He devised an exercise to enable pupils to achieve this. He taught them to breathe out on a whispered 'ah'. (This has since become one of the cornerstones of Alexander lessons). Once pupils have learned to do this, they do not put undue strain on the vocal cords.

The toll of 'civilisation'

At the time Alexander was writing and teaching, Freud's theories about the unconscious mind became enthusiastically adopted by many contemporary intellectuals, but not by FM. He did not believe that the conscious and unconscious minds could be separated as Freudians asserted. Rather, he believed that conscious and subconscious acts are part of the same process.

We start off, he said, by doing things consciously. Then constant repetition of the same act renders it unconscious and outside ordinary control. Habits are acquired below the level of the conscious mind, and yet we can make conscious attempts to rid ourselves of them. Alexander did not believe in hypnotism, mesmerism or attempts to probe the unconscious mind. He felt these were all unnecessary and could even be dangerous – they might winkle out the wrong habit without replacing it with a good one. He argued that nature abhors a vacuum. Therefore it is not possible simply to remove a bad habit. It will only go away when something better, and equally ingrained, is put in its place.

So how, it may be asked, did we get like this? How is it that humans have become largely creatures of bad habits? Why haven't we developed good ones instead? The answer, for Alexander, lay in the effects of evolution and 'civilisation': Man has ceased to be a natural animal and lives in a largely artificial environment. We spend most of our time sitting in chairs, driving around in cars and at offices or in homes which are far removed from anything intended by nature.

Also, we are no longer dependent on the physical body for our existence. We do not have to walk to get around, we do not usually have to run away from danger, and we do not even have to keep ourselves physically fit in order to function. Indeed, in the modern world it is possible to function without using the body at all. So, over the centuries, we have lost our ability to be natural with our bodies, and have long forgotten what natural, harmonious movement is. The resultant imbalances can lead to serious illnesses, but if you give back to the body its natural functioning, then conditions are created for good, lasting health.

Even so, Alexander was not in the ordinary sense of the word, a 'primitive', back to nature kind of man. He enjoyed the benefits of civilisation, such as good food and drink, and was somewhat addicted to horse racing.

His busy schedule and voluminous writings did not leave much time for family life. In 1920 he married Edith Page, an actress, but the marriage was not happy, and for much of their lives they lived apart. Her antagonism to him became so great that she would not allow their adopted daughter to take Alexander lessons. In later years, Alexander discreetly acquired a mistress and a son.

A famous patient

During the 1930s, Alexander's work was popularised by Aldous Huxley, who had suffered from various illnesses since childhood. In later life, Huxley also became plagued by periods of deep depression. When he consulted FM, he was told that this was mainly due to his attitudes while writing, and self-enforced long periods of concentration. Alexander believed that nobody should concentrate on one piece of work for more than an hour-and-a-half at a time. During periods of deep mental concentration, it was all too easy to forget about posture, breathing and all the other physical acts which could eventually lead to bad usage. Therefore he advised a short break for 10 minutes or so, and a conscious effort to realign the body.

If these breaks were not taken, mental and physical problems would soon threaten to stop the flow of concentration anyway. Concentration would actually have turned into stress and anxiety, and be counter-productive.

Once Huxley understood the theory, he lost no time in explaining it in his novels. In *Eyeless in Gaza*, Huxley's hero Anthony Beavis explains Miller's (Alexander's) philosophy:

> *Miller says of age that it's largely a matter of habit. Use conditions function. Walk about as if you were a martyr to rheumatism and you'll impose such violent muscular strains upon yourself that a martyr to rheumatism you'll really be. Behave like an old man and your body will function like an old man's, you'll think and feel as an old man. The lean and slippered pantaloon – largely a part that one plays. If you refuse to play it and learn to act on your refusal, you won't become a pantaloon.*

Huxley accepted Alexander's theory that mind and body are essentially one, and that whatever goes on inside the head is communicated to the body, and vice versa, so that even everyday, seemingly trivial actions are, in fact, important. This means we must become conscious again of *everything* we do, even to the way we tie our shoelaces or shut a door, as these will eventually affect the way we think and behave.

For example, we may clench our fists when we are angry, hunch our shoulders when afraid, twitch and fiddle when nervous. In time these actions can become part of us, and influence the functioning of our bodies and our minds. And the way we use our bodies can actually affect what we become. If we walk around as though we are confident and self-assured, our bodies will receive this message, and in time we will actually become self-confident. If, conversely, we walk around in a nervous, tense manner, that is what we will become.

Huxley's Anthony Beavis explains how he feels after attending a lesson with Miller:

> *At today's lesson with Miller found myself suddenly a step forward in my grasp of the theory and practice of the technique. To learn proper use one must first inhibit all improper uses of the self. Refuse to be hurried into gaining ends by the equivalent (in psycho-physiological terms) of violent revolution; inhibit this tendency and concentrate on the means whereby this end is to be achieved; then act. This process*

*entails knowing good and bad use – knowing them apart. By the
'feel', increased awareness and increased power of control result.*

This passage introduces us to another famous Alex-
anderism – the notion of *inhibition*, here having a completely
different meaning from that understood by Freudians. In
Alexander language, inhibition is a good thing – you consciously inhibit bad actions and learn to replace them by good
ones. You learn to think before you act, in every situation.

Alexander taught that if you concentrate on the correct use
of the body you will automatically transfer such correct use to
the mind. As Huxley observed you can also inhibit more
complicated trains of behaviour. The neurotic and the luna-
tic, he continued, are both characterised by their stooping,
sad, resigned posture. If they can be encouraged to walk
upright, according to the theory, they will eventually then lose
their neuroticism and their lunacy. When you substitute a bad
habit for a good one, you are then giving the mind a new set of
instructions.

The later years

Although Alexander consolidated his reputation in Britain
during the 1930s, when war broke out again in 1939 he sailed
to America. On his return to England in 1943 he discovered
that criticism of his work was growing. He was incensed by a
scathing attack on his work published in South Africa – where
his reputation had been extremely high – by a Dr Ernst Jokl, a
South African physical education teacher. A court case followed, which Alexander won.

Although by now well into his seventies, Alexander continued to teach for around 16 hours a day. He was seemingly
inexhaustible, and put his superabundant energy down to
practising what he preached. But in 1947 when he was 79, he
suffered a stroke which temporarily cost him the use of one leg
and one arm, and the left side of his face became paralysed.
Remarkably he recovered and continued to teach until his
death, on October 10, 1955, after a short illness. He was 86.
During his last years, he had continued refining his method,
and trained other teachers to carry on his work.

Yet, for all his achievements, Frederick Matthias Alexander is not a household name in the same way that, say, Freud and Jung are. American Alexander teacher Michael Gelb, author of the book *Body Learning*, believes there are two reasons for this. One is that Alexander never became part of the 'establishment' and, all his life, continued to fall out with influential people. He was also extremely reluctant to delegate, or – until his later years – to pass on his teachings. He felt that he was the only one who could properly teach The Method.

Because he trained so few teachers, things went very quiet from when he died, on through the sixties. In Britain, his work was kept alive mainly by Wilfred Barlow, a doctor who married into Alexander's family, and combined teaching the technique with his more conventional medical practice.

Method scientifically proved

Only when academics at one or two American universities decided to put the Alexander Technique to scientific investigation did the method begin to be revived, and gradually achieve the popularity it enjoys today.

Using strobostrobic photography and electromyography (equipment not invented in Alexander's day) they were able to demonstrate that the movements, and 'use' of the body that Alexander taught did have far-reaching positive effects. He had indeed discovered a technique whereby bad habits could be relinquished and better ones substituted.

It was proved beyond all possible doubt that the Technique was not just an airy-fairy placebo, but actually did work and could benefit around 99 per cent of the population.

Further studies in America showed that, by the age of 11, the vast majority of children's bodies are already quite seriously out of alignment, and set on a wrong path that may eventually, if not corrected, cause mental, emotional and physical problems.

With the renewed interest in all methods of alternative medicine, and in the holistic approach, which seeks to unify body, mind and spirit, Alexander's work is at last getting the recognition it deserves. As more people are finding that high-tech, drug-based medicine is failing them, they are turning in ever increasing numbers to alternative therapies.

The Alexander method demands a fundamental revision in the way we conduct ourselves and think of ourselves. It demands practice, hard work and a good teacher. Luckily, there are now many excellent Alexander teachers available, who can pass on to others Alexander's valuable lessons.

2

The Technique explained

Even many teachers and practitioners hesitate to give a concise definition of the Alexander Technique, and prefer to tell you what it is *not* rather than what it is.

It is not exactly relaxation, they will tell you, nor is it a set of physical exercises. Nor does it consist of actually learning anything. Rather, it is a way of unlearning how you already, wrongly, use your body. And as the things we are doing wrong with our bodies have probably become ingrained habits, it is not just a matter of saying: do this from now on, and you will feel better.

To complicate matters further, Alexander employed terms such as 'primary control', 'use', 'endgaining', 'means-whereby' and 'inhibition', which he used in a special sense to describe what humans do to themselves.

But once the underlying principles are understood and the jargon explained, the Technique is not difficult to understand, to teach or to put into practice.

Above all, Alexander believed that most of us put far too much effort into ordinary everyday tasks, such as bending down, sitting, standing or walking. Furthermore, we often contort our bodies into unnatural shapes and positions, usually without realising it. A small child, he said, naturally walks correctly and with proper use of the spine. In a very short time, however, this same child will develop bad posture, and bad 'use' of the body. The child learns this bad use by imitation of adults, and by being told wrongly how to do things by these same adults.

These learned bad habits are reinforced further by sitting in badly-designed chairs, and by negative emotional reactions to stimuli. Excessive shyness or fear can easily cause bad posture in quite a young child. At the same time as the body will pick up wrong ways of 'use', so the mind will start to acquire bad, or negative ways of thinking. Gradually, these habits of standing, speaking and so on become so ingrained that they are actually part of us, 'our' way of doing things. It all happens so subtly and so unconsciously that nobody notices – least of all the individual who is developing the wrong habits.

The whole essence of the Alexander method is to demonstrate new and better ways of moving, so that new habits can drive out the old. And the earlier in life this can be done, the easier it will be.

Most children do not know, and are never taught, the right ways of sitting, standing, breathing and even talking. They are not taught because their teachers themselves do not know. But wrong ways of conducting ourselves physically have a cumulative effect, as they put excess strain on muscles and joints. By the time most of us are young adults, the spine will be right out of alignment, and this will set up problems in all joints, including those in the legs and feet. Whatever affects the spine will in time affect the vital organs, so wrong posture and wrong sitting positions can also lead to heart, kidney and lung trouble in later life.

If the body is helped gently and expertly back into its proper alignment, we notice more than physical benefits. Old ways of thinking and emotions clear and we can develop a new optimism, confidence and calmness. Through concentrating entirely on the body, and forgetting about the mind, we can rid ourselves of all kinds of negative attitudes which may be hindering both mental and physical health.

Negative influences

The big question is: since we are all at birth endowed with a spine which is perfectly capable of doing its job without strain and sprain, why should we start to pick up bad habits so early in life, habits which are simply not noticed by us or those around us?

It starts mainly in schools, Alexander believed. All of his life, he inveighed against modern educational methods, believing that they did far more harm than good. In primitive tribes, he said, children do not go to school, but play around the village compound in blissful ignorance of books and classrooms. Nowadays, children have to go to school by law and – with very few exceptions – spend the largest part of their childhood in a mixture of boredom and fear. In most children, stated Alexander, the boredom they experience leads them to slump in their chairs and over their desks, and to slouch at every opportunity.

Television was in its infancy in Alexander's day, but

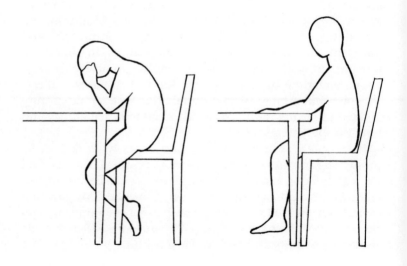

Child slumped at desk   *A more poised sitting position*

modern Alexander teachers say that it worsens the problems. After slumping and slouching all day in chairs, children come home and slump in front of the television.

Ordinary physical education lessons cannot right this misuse. Alexander felt that, on the whole, school physical education programmes were more concerned with winning cups and breaking records, than interested in the individual child's correct physical growth. Some Alexander teachers now consider that the more highly trained children are in sports and athletics, the more liable they are to experience physical problems in later life. This happens because many sports coaches and instructors rarely pause to consider what they might be doing to a youngster's body when they encourage him or her to concentrate on breaking records or winning ever more matches.

Young gymnasts, for instance, spend most of their childhood practising, in order to reach international standard by the age of 14 or 15. The constant practising demanded by today's almost impossibly high standards means that their bodies will have become permanently deformed by the time they reach early adolescence. The same happens to promising tennis players, swimmers, athletes and dancers. As most such activities require the body to be twisted into unnatural positions, sometimes for hours on end, it is not surprising that in time, all joints and muscles will be out of alignment.

Indeed, since such activities have become fiercely competitive, the number of serious injuries suffered by young people has soared. Many doctors specialise in treating such injuries, and there is hardly an international player of any sport who has not sustained major injuries. Young tennis player Tracy Austin, a child prodigy, had to give up the game in her early twenties because of repeated, bad injuries caused by over-practising. The same happened to Andrea Jaeger, again an international tennis player in her early teens. Billie Jean King, six times women's singles winner at Wimbledon, has permanently damaged her knee joints through the heavy demands of international tennis. The point is, in Alexander terms, if one damages a knee, or other joint, this will inevitably affect other joints. This is because everything in the body is interconnected, nothing works in isolation.

Muscle tears, hip diseases, Achilles tendon pain, torn hamstrings, are all conditions resulting from overuse of a very small group of muscles. In later life, these injuries can lead to rheumatism and arthritis, gout and the need for hip replacement operations. Far from making people fit, modern sports programmes tend to 'unfit' them for health in later life.

Alexander teachers are not against sport, or dancing, and they are certainly not in favour of being unfit. The trouble is, most athletes and dancers are taught only to think about the end result. They hardly ever pause to consider, in Alexander terms, the 'means-whereby'. Yet, if more attention was paid to the means, it would be possible for far more people to enjoy these activities throughout their lives, and so keep themselves healthy and fit.

Physical deformities do not have to be great to cause ill-health. Even the habit of crossing your legs when sitting down will, over the years, put the body quite seriously out of alignment. If your job entails a lot of telephoning, the way you answer the telephone can cause your neck to become out of alignment with your head and body. Even such apparently small things can set up imbalances in the body severe enough to cause actual illness.

But it is always possible to correct the deformities – at least to an extent which will be beneficial – by learning and practising the Alexander Technique. So, here is a brief guide to the main Alexander concepts:

Primary control

By this, Alexander meant the relationship of the head and neck to the rest of the body. If that is right, then the rest of the body will be properly aligned.

In most of us, this is not the case; we tend to throw back the head and stiffen and shorten the spine when sitting down. We are, of course, completely unaware that we are doing this – and do it all the time. Eventually, the spine curves and can no longer become upright, however much we try. One can see the end result of years of misuse in the badly curved spines and dowager's humps of many old people.

This apparent problem of old age actually starts in youth,

and very often, in childhood. If we habitually pull back the skull on sitting down, sooner or later we will experience lower back pain. We are hardly ever aware, though, that we are pulling our heads back unnecessarily. By habitually moving in certain ways, says leading Alexander teacher Wilfred Barlow, 'we begin to alter our physique.'

One way to regain correct 'primary control' is to imagine at all times that there is a cord coming out of the top of your head and pulling you gently towards the sky. This will enable you to lengthen and widen the spine, which is essential for correct posture and balance. Practise it now, and all through the day. It will help your body to go back into its proper alignment, and give all organs and muscles a chance to get back into their proper place.

When sitting down, the great majority of people pull their heads back onto their shoulders and arch their backs. This can lead to a condition known as lordosis, in which the spine has become permanently curved and is noticed as a 'hollow back'.

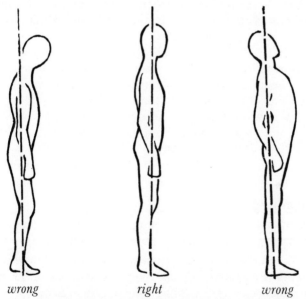

wrong   *right*   *wrong*

Directing the head forward and up helps the body to find an easier alignment

Getting the 'primary control' correct is important, not only for posture, grace and ease of movement, but also for brain function. If we cannot get fully and properly upright, we spoil our chances of achieving our full potential, both mentally and physically. The Alexander Technique teaches you how to lengthen the muscles in your spine, so that a properly upright position can be maintained. One of the first benefits of practising this lesson is that pressure is relieved on the discs between the bones of the spine, and there is an increase in height.

Getting the primary control right means that we can start to become conscious of the way we move, stand and sit down. Most people who have been for Alexander lessons notice that, as posture improves, attitudes also alter for the better and mental tensions and anxieties disperse.

Antigravity

The gravity response means that everything is continually being pulled downwards. Alexander believed that we consciously have to fight against this tendency and invoke the 'antigravity' response instead. This means paying continuous attention to lengthening the spine at every opportunity, and always being aware of that invisible string pulling skywards. Do not look up, but imagine that the cord is coming from the top of your head. If this is practised constantly, there will be a feeling of lightness and grace in every movement, and backaches, head and neck problems will cease to exist.

'Endgaining'

This is another very important Alexander concept. The great majority of people are so keen on achieving the end result that they completely forget to pay any attention to how they set about doing a particular task. When we sit down, for example, most of us never give a thought as to how we change from a standing position to a sitting one. All we know is that suddenly we are sitting down. We may consider that the act of sitting down is a trivial action, but for Alexander there is no such thing. Every action that causes an alteration of bodily position is important.

Usually, we use an unnecessary and inappropriate amount of tension to achieve our end, and in our eagerness to achieve it, most of us never stop to think about whether the means we are employing may be harmful. For Alexander, the end never justified the means – it was always the means that were most important.

Endgaining is one of the most original and revolutionary of all the Alexander concepts. When we endgain, he said, we always employ over-quick and over-energetic means. The idea is that the goal should be achieved as quickly as possible, so that we can move on to the next one. If we are endgainers in one thing, Alexander argued, we will be endgainers in everything. We will be over hasty in eating food, opening doors, driving a car or making sure that our views are heard.

Endgaining is at its most pernicious in schools. Children are taught that only the results, the exam passes, matter, so that they can enter the next stage, where there will be more exams, more hurdles to cross. Such pressures produce those who have been defined as 'Type A' people, hell-bent on success at any terms, even including heart attacks and agonising back pain. These are the typical endgainers.

It should not be thought that Alexander was against achievement. Far from it. He was himself an achiever, but he felt that endgaining principles stored up long-term troubles, by going for the short-term satisfaction, rather than paying attention to long-term possible disbenefits.

The process of 'endgaining' is, as Alexander saw it, endemic to our society. When we are ill, we go to the doctor for a pill which is supposed to resolve the problem. We want immediate answers and solutions. In the same way, artificial fertilisers are sprayed on to crops to get bigger, better and more reliable harvests. But all the time, the earth is becoming impoverished, and each year, an increasing amount of artificial fertiliser is sprayed on to achieve the same results.

While we employ the 'endgaining' approach, we are not giving any thought to the means we employ to reach our desired goal. But if we can only slow down and think instead about the means, there is a good chance that bodily functions will begin to right themselves.

The 'means-whereby'

This term refers to the ways in which we do things, the means employed to achieve the end. Instead of merely thinking about what we want to achieve, we ought to consider our motivations, our abilities, and our suitability for particular tasks.

Learning to concentrate on the 'means-whereby' will enable us to correct long-ingrained bad habits. It is no use saying to somebody who slumps, 'Stand up straight.' He or she may pull themselves up temporarily, but will always naturally return to the slumping position. The only way to correct a slump is to monitor carefully what you are doing every time you stand up. Gradually, by paying attention to the various stages of standing up, bad postural habits will be corrected. Only when you are able to feel the difference for yourself, will you gain conscious control.

Whenever we do things wrongly – and according to Alexander, endgainers will always set about doing things wrongly – we encourage wrong habits to become more ingrained. In sport, this process is called 'grooving'. Sports coaches know that every time the player hits a ball wrongly, this increases the chances of him doing it again. The only way to correct the action is to go back to basics. Sports psychologists – who are now becoming as important as sports coaches – try to find out why the ball is being hit wrongly, and why a wrong swing has developed. In most cases, this will be due to fear, anxiety and tension.

Learning to forget about the end result, learning not to let it matter, reduces stress and tension in body and mind. Whenever we concentrate on the means, we allow the end to happen naturally. The process is basically one of learning inner calm, so that self-confidence and self-esteem can develop.

Inhibition

The way Alexander used this word is not to be confused with

30

the Freudian term. In the Technique, 'inhibition' means that you learn to stop, or consciously 'inhibit' bad actions.

Alexander believed that it was impossible to inhibit bad actions by willpower alone, by telling yourself not to do something. The only possible way of driving out a wrong habit is gradually to substitute a good one. It is no good saying to yourself, 'I will not hunch my shoulders,' as most of the time you will not even be aware that you are hunching your shoulders. But if you order yourself to lengthen your spine, and widen it out, your shoulders will stop hunching; you will 'inhibit' the bad action which leads to body asymmetry and deformity.

This inhibiting has nothing to do with repressing natural emotions or reactions. It is a means of stopping the endgaining response which, in most people, eventually becomes a reflex action that bypasses the conscious brain. The process of inhibiting allows this same action to come back into the realms of conscious activity, so that it is no longer reflex. It is the reflex, automatic actions which do the damage.

Learning to inhibit wrong actions may be quite slow and laborious depending on how ingrained they have become. Next time you get dressed, stop and consider which sock you usually put on first. Have you any idea? Most of us haven't any notion of the order in which we get dressed. It is only when we can no longer carry out these reflex actions, for some reason, such as if we break an arm, that we are forced to consider how we do things.

When we learn to give ourselves orders before we do things puts unconscious actions back into the conscious control, and enables us to exert more power and forethought. We do things 'unconsciously' when we are so used to doing them that our minds are elsewhere. Most people are not concentrating on getting dressed in the morning, but are worrying about work, and the day ahead generally.

None of this would matter if we performed these unconscious, reflex actions correctly. The chances are, though, that we do not, and that every time we put our socks on, we twist our bodies into unnatural shapes.

Learn to inhibit the reflexes, both body and mind are given a new dynamism and strength.

Use

This refers to the way in which we use (or more commonly, misuse) our bodies. The theory behind the Alexander Technique states that personality, character and emotions are all intimately affected by the ways in which we use our bodies.

Alexander worked out that the main reason for his own recurring voice problem was persistent misuse of his body (see Chapter One). When correcting misuse generally, the first aim must be to regain proper use of the head and neck, the 'primary control'. From that, all other use follows.

Once we regain good use, then our potential for achievement becomes limitless, said Alexander. The best use is that which promotes the most efficient functioning of the human system, and enables us to regain correct balance. Once the body is correctly balanced, then all kinds of tension-related disorders, such as migraine, lower back pain, stomach ulcers, can correct themselves. Correct use involves re-educating the muscles to move in different ways.

Function

This word refers to the ways in which the body works. All of our organs, limbs and muscles have specific functions, and work in a certain way. When we employ wrong use this interferes with the function, and body organs cannot work as they should. Correct use restores proper function.

Stimulus

This is a favourite Alexander word, to describe whatever sets off a specific type of movement. Through constantly-repeated habits, the kinds of movement activated by a particular function become automatic. We have to re-educate ourselves to become aware of all the stimuli – mental, physical and emotional – which set off a particular set of reactions.

We can alter our response to stimuli. In fact, all responses can come within our conscious control. For example, we may feel we can't help being angry when somebody lets us down, or displeases us in some way. In fact, the anger and the hurt have become a learned response, another habit.

Our bodies, also, respond in automatic ways – if we are not careful. We may imagine that trembling, twitching, stuttering, are involuntary movements. In fact, we learned them – so long ago that they seem always to have been with us. People suffering from a serious disability such as Parkinson's Disease may not be able to control their limbs, but most of us can, if we want to, learn to alter our response to all stimuli.

The whole purpose of Alexander teaching is to bring more of life into our conscious control, so that in a very real way we become masters of our fate. Altering our set reaction to stimuli frees both body and mind from being narrowly channelled.

Above all, learning the Alexander methods means you have to be prepared to let go of your attachment to the past, to let go of old, outdated responses and replace them with new, dynamic ways of thinking and acting. It is hanging on to the past, in the form of ingrained habits, which blights our future. Learn to let it go – and the 'real' you emerges.

3

The physical benefits

Above all, the Alexander Technique consists of understanding what the founder termed 'primary control' – that is, the relationship of the head and neck in relation to the rest of the body. Once that is in alignment, then the rest of the body will necessarily be maintained in good shape. The problem is, most people tend to throw the head and neck back and stiffen and shorten the spine when changing position from standing to sitting.

Alexander paid particular attention to the spine, because he felt this was where all major health problems started. One reason for this is that most people have no idea whatever how the spinal column works, and how the head, neck and body relate to each other. He believed that though we have been well-designed by nature, our modern environment tended to distort and deform our upright position, and that negative emotions such as fear, anxiety and anger further worked against a naturally balanced physical position.

Unlike many other animals, humans possess necks which are very free to move, and which give a very useful wide range of vision. But the disadvantage of a freely-moving neck is that we are free to move it in the wrong ways. A long neck, says leading Alexander teacher Wilfred Barlow, gives humans more freedom of movement, but also means that more muscle groups than are strictly necessary can be used. This is one reason why we tend to put far too much energy and effort into everyday tasks. If we observe domestic animals such as cats and dogs, we will see that they never expend useless energy. Nor do most wild animals. Humans are the only creatures who habitually over-use certain muscle groups – and that is why back and spinal problems are so common. Whenever muscles are used unnecessarily, undue strain is put on the back and spinal cord.

We even use too many muscles in speaking, swallowing and breathing. This can lead to important muscles in the head and neck becoming locked. The Alexander Technique helps people to regain freedom of the head and neck by teaching a new system of balance, specifically developed to promote the most effective use of the muscles.

Alexander balance differs from that which most people ordinarily adopt, as the centre of gravity is much further back. Instead of sloping forward and humping the back, causing a large hollow at the waist and a protruding stomach, the pupil is taught to maintain as straight a line as possible all the way down the back. Instead of the bones in the neck being allowed to drop forward and downward, they are asked to go upward and back. This does not mean adopting a rigid stiff-upper-lip, military-type bearing, but being relaxed and unrigid through-out the body. Once this is achieved, muscle tension in the neck and lower back is immediately released, and height increases slightly.

Another important aspect of the Alexander principle is that the knees are not locked rigidly, but are very slightly bent, with the thighs a little apart. This type of balance enables each vertebra in the back to move separately, rather than being contracted and locked. Pressure is instantly relieved on the fluid-filled discs between the vertebrae, and they can start to expand. This is a major reason for the feeling of increased lightness and antigravity which most Alexander pupils soon start to observe.

Most important of all, Alexander developed a way of stand-ing which meant that the whole body – shoulders, elbows, hands, hips, knees, ankles and feet – remained in a position whereby all the joint surfaces lengthened away from each other, rather than being shortened. (Every time we sit, stand or walk in a cramped position, we shorten the muscles.)

Recent research by exercise physiologists has confirmed

that the important aspect of muscle balance *is* lengthening, rather than shortening. Most warm-up exercises are designed to lengthen muscles and keep them that way. In most of us, muscles are constantly being shortened: sitting in so-called comfortable chairs, in offices or homes, driving cars and travelling on buses and aeroplanes all shorten muscles.

When an Alexander teacher asks a pupil to squat, often this position – which comes so easily to children – will prove impossible for the pupil to perform. Over the years, the muscles have seized up to such an extent that they can no longer get into the correct positions. The main reason why the average person cannot sit cross-legged or in the yoga Lotus Position for very long is because the muscles have become too short. In Eastern countries, where squatting is the standard form of sitting, and chairs are in short supply, this ability is retained into old age.

When most people sit down, they contract the head on to the shoulders, arch the back and thrust their bottoms out. This also shortens muscles and contracts the spine. So, instead of just plonking yourself into a chair, bend your knees and then slowly lower yourself into the chair, letting your knees rather than your back do the work. Then the pelvis will not push back, and the chest will not come forward. Most people have got so used to merely flopping down that they find it difficult to sit down in the 'proper' way.

The knees should never be crossed, but pointed away from each other; crossed knees inhibit the circulation and, more importantly, increase the likelihood of developing lower back pain. Anybody whose job involves sitting for long hours should keep checking to make sure their knees are not crossed.

As Wilfred Barlow points out in his book, *The Alexander Principle*, the technique is not just one man's idiosyncratic ideas. The Alexander method not only restores spinal and muscular balance, but actually alters what goes on inside the head. All variations on pressure felt throughout the body are immediately registered in the skull. Information is conveyed more accurately through the complicated bio-chemical channels if the head is balanced properly on the neck. This means that the head's own 'spirit-level' is properly balanced.

The spine

An appreciation of the Alexander Technique starts with an understanding of the spine. Here is a simplified version of what the spine does, when working properly.

It has four main functions:

- To give the support necessary for humans to maintain an upright posture.

- To protect the spinal cord and network of nerves emanating from it.

- To allow a wide range of movements but at the same time prevent damage to the body.

- To connect the head, shoulders, pelvis and legs.

The spinal cord is made up of a large number of bones called the vertebrae. These are separated and cushioned by oval pads known as discs. There are 33 vertebrae, contained in five separate sections of the spine. They are shaped like a drum and have an upright tube attached to the back. This drum is positioned so that its flat surfaces are at the top and bottom. The vertebrae encircle the body's main nerve pathways, and are held in place by many different muscles.

The spine is not straight; it curves in three places. First there is the cervical curve, in the neck. Then comes the thoracic curve, at the rib cage and, finally, the lumbar curve in the lower back. The lumbar curve, particularly, brings the centre of gravity down over the legs, and exerts a downward force on the hip bones.

Each vertebra is connected to the one below, and this enables the whole spine to be extremely flexible. Greater flexibility of the spine can be achieved with regular practice, as yogis and gymnasts discover. But just as the spine can become more flexible, so it can also become extremely rigid. It is also quite easy for the delicately-balanced vertebral connections to be wrenched out of position by wrong posture, slumping and wrong methods of sitting.

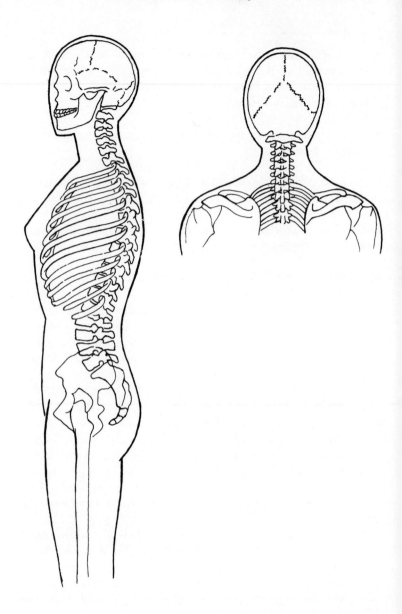

The vertebrae

The shape of the spine alters throughout our lifetime – naturally. It is meant to. Newborn infants have a C-shaped spinal cord, and this gradually elongates to the S-shape in adolescence and adulthood. As the body ages, the discs between the vertebrae lose some of their sponginess by chemical dehydration. The Alexander Technique can to some extent prevent this 'squashing down' of the discs which is mainly responsible for the loss of height in many people over the age of 60.

The first vertebra, at the top of the neck, is known as the atlas. This ring of bone supports the skull and contents of the head. It interlocks with the second vertebra, known as the axis, which has a bony projection at the top, on which the atlas pivots, enabling us to turn our heads. Then we have five more cervical vertebrae which are very similar to each other.

Each vertebra has several bony projections. If we run our hands down our backs, we can feel these. Each vertebra links on to the next by means of one of these bones, and the others form attachments for the many muscles in the back.

The next group is the 12 thoracic vertebrae. Some connect with the ribs, and form the joints which allow our chests to expand as we breathe. Below these are the five lumbar vertebrae which, with the muscles attached to them, support our body weight. The spinal cord runs only as far as the lumbar vertebrae, and then becomes a tiny string as it goes into the next five vertebrae, known as the sacrum. This forms the back wall of the pelvis.

At the bottom of the spine are the final five vertebrae which make up the coccyx, or tail bone.

Attached to all these vertebrae are more than 80 muscles in and around the neck alone. The muscles are of three main groups, and all connect up with other muscles in the body. Thus, the head, neck and back constitute the nerve centre of the body. Any tension, mental ·or physical, is instantly referred to the back.

Common spinal problems

Thanks to the two main vertebrae in the neck – the atlas and the axis – the head can rotate through an angle of 180 degrees.

This allows much freedom of movement, but at the same time it means that there is always a lot of wear and tear on these vertebrae and the discs between them. If the spine in the neck region is subject to too much wear and tear, then narrowing of the spaces through which nerve roots pass can occur. This results in pain felt in the neck, shoulder, elbow and even fingers. This condition is known as cervical spondylosis, and the usual treatment is to wear a surgical collar to stop the head from being rotated too far. This can clear up the problem in the short term, but if we persist in using our necks wrongly, the condition will always be liable to recur.

The thoracic area is less likely to cause problems because movements here are fairly restricted, owing to the need to provide stability to vital organs such as the heart and lungs.

By far the great majority of problems occur in the lower back, which takes the weight of the whole body, plus anything extra that may be carried. Most bending that we do takes place in this area. As this part of the spine takes most of the wear and tear, it is particularly liable to injury. According to physiotherapist Christopher Hayne, author of *Total Back Care*, around 85 per cent of spinal problems occur in this part of the body.

He goes on to say that anybody over the age of 50 is almost certain to have degenerative changes in the fifth lumbar disc, and also probably in the third and fourth lumbar discs. Alexander would say that these changes are almost certainly caused by wrong use, repeated hundreds or thousands of times in the past 50 years.

The muscles

There are three main groups of muscles attached to the bones of the spinal cord – at the back, at the front and at the sides of the spine – and these too, are very important.

The basic function of the spinal muscles is to counteract the effects of gravity, and to keep the trunk stable. Whenever the spine bends forward, the large spinal muscles in the lumbar region have to work harder. This places stress on the ligaments which stretch to take the increased load. Whenever we bend, or pick up a load incorrectly, a huge amount of strain is placed on these ligaments. As most of us bend, stoop and lift things many times in each day, the strain on the back muscles may be very great.

Back doctors now understand the need for lengthy rest periods – something which Alexander also advocated. He reasoned that if we used muscles incorrectly, we were unable to rest them properly. This is why he formulated his theory of 'resting balance', and emphasised the need for economy of effort. The less undue effort we put into all physical tasks, the less will be the strain on important muscles in the back.

We have to learn to stop making muscular contractions when we rest. Alexander devised a way of lying down which would promote deep relaxation and rest – but we have to make ourselves do it every day otherwise there will not be any appreciable benefits. He said that if we could teach ourselves to lie down on the floor, our head resting on a sufficient number of books to bring our head into a normal relationship to the body and with the back no longer arched, then the muscles would have a good chance of regaining their elasticity and stretch.

When muscles are used wrongly, they shorten and lose elasticity. Unfortunately, they will not readily regain their proper length by ordinary rest, or stopping whatever activity made them shorten in the first place. But they can return to their proper resting length by Alexander-type body learning.

When muscles are used in wrong ways, they continue to be in a state of activity even when their owners are doing nothing. Something has gone wrong with the feedback mechanism to the brain, which has not registered the fact that the muscle has stopped working. The contraction continues, and muscles may go into spasm, or twitch.

Continual misuse of muscles sets in when we have no idea how to return to a properly balanced resting state in which the muscles can become relaxed and go back to their proper length. In time, says Wilfred Barlow, the resting state of the muscle not only becomes wrongly balanced, but starts to affect the bones and joints to which it is joined. The bones can become warped and out of shape due to the strains placed on them by persistent over-contraction of the muscle. Over the years, muscular over-contraction can cause the whole body to become deformed so that it can never return to its proper resting state.

As we get older, it is likely that our bodies will return to an ever more unbalanced resting state, so that stress remains in the system after physical activity. The residual muscular tension shows itself up in lower back pains, headaches, neuralgia, lumbago and aches and pains in the knees and legs. This happens because the body can no longer become perfectly relaxed, even when asleep. 'Tension', says Wilfred Barlow, 'remains latent in an unbalanced resting state.' By this stage, only a process of unlearning and then re-learning by conscious attention can direct the body into a more balanced position.

How the Alexander Technique can help

The Alexander Technique teaches people to expel all the tension held in the body when it is supposed to be at rest. It really is a way of learning how to rest, so that the body can return to normal. Whenever somebody is suffering from residual tension, it becomes impossible to relax the muscles completely, and injuries can result.

Common kinds of back pain include **soft tissue injuries**, which develop when there is prolonged over-use and strain. They can develop during activities such as sports, dancing, gardening, and do-it-yourself work. These injuries are especially likely to develop when there is a history of poor posture or tension – or long exposure to cold.

Soft tissue injuries are confined to muscles and ligaments. They often begin with a sharp pain, which may eventually become a dull ache or chronic tenderness. Connective tissues may have become torn, and caused swelling or bleeding in the area. Very often, it is possible to activate the pain by touching a particular spot. Doctors often call this condition 'fibrositis'.

Injuries concerning the **ligaments** also happen to people who habitually sit, stand or walk badly. The damage is cumulative and may not be noticed for many years, as ligaments are extremely tough. When they tear, though, they tend to heal slowly. When the back is habitually rounded, rather than straight, this causes the ligaments to stretch unnaturally and become deformed.

This kind of injury is characterised by acute pain, followed by swelling. After resting, there may be residual ache which never really goes away, and is felt as chronic aches and fatigue. If the posture can be corrected according to Alexander principles, healing can take place.

'Slipped disc'

There is really no such condition as a 'slipped disc', as discs cannot slip between vertebrae. The correct medical term for this condition is Prolapsed Intervertebral Disc, or PID. What happens, is that the disc gradually loses its shock-absorbing capacities and becomes flat and crushed. The main reason for this is undue stress in the lumbar region. It used to be thought that 'slipped discs' were almost an inevitable part of getting older but, as Alexander understood, it is really poor posture and accumulated stress on the spine which causes the discs to collapse. There is no anatomical reason for them to slip in older people.

The severe pain which sufferers experience is caused by degeneration of the chemical structure of the disc, which causes its fibres to crack and burst apart. Then the central nucleus can rupture and enter the vertebral canal, where it presses on the nerve root. This is the stage at which bad pain is felt, although the damage has probably been there for years.

PID happens mainly in older people as in the teens and early twenties the discs are strong enough to resist the forces that may be applied to them, even when these constitute wrong use. Over a long period of misuse, however, the disc becomes unable to withstand the unnatural strain.

The usual treatment advocated for slipped discs is plenty of rest, keeping warm, and taking painkillers. This allows the inflammation to subside, and the cracks to seal up. It may take up to three months for full recovery to be achieved, and unless habits are changed, the condition will eventually recur.

Chronic back pain

Low-grade, persistent backache is very common. In fact, it is one of the commonest reasons for people taking days off work.

Like the other back problems, it is caused by long-term changes in the vertebrae and tissues. Whenever parts of the spine are out of alignment, there is a danger that excess strain on other parts will lead eventually to chronic pain. Sitting and standing in a poor position, doing work which involves a lot of bending, will cause back pain to develop. A healthy, straight back can withstand long periods of standing or sitting. A faulty back cannot.

Back pain is by far the commonest reason for people to seek out Alexander teachers. Unlike medical doctors, they will not ask you to take your clothes off, or examine you in any formal way. They do not, like chiropractors, take X-rays of the affected area. They do not need to – they already know what has brought their patients to such a sorry plight. This is years of bad back use.

Case History – Helen Dasquez

Helen Dasquez, a teacher and farmer, became incapacitated with severe back pains. She said: 'I went to my doctor, and it was found I had lost elasticity in the lumbar region. I had several X-rays and then went to see a specialist who said there was nothing for it but to take steroids.

'After that I visited an osteopath, who said I had severe muscular damage and was doing too much. Apart from running a farm and teaching, I also look after horses – and knew I was doing far too much. But it wasn't easy to stop any of it. I knew my posture wasn't good and never had been, but had no idea how to improve it.

'Then I saw a TV programme about the Alexander Technique and thought it sounded just right. I had a lesson and for the very first time in my life I experienced benefit, though it was two years before my back righted itself.

'I realise now that if you damage the muscles they will take a long time to go back to normal. Also, if you use your body wrongly, this can only aggravate the damage. This was why my problem was getting worse all the time. Now, I practise the Alexander Technique daily, and can do all the heavy jobs I couldn't manage before, such as the stable work, riding, and looking after the horses.'

Like many other people, **Helen Dasquez** had 'tried everything' before taking Alexander lessons. Aged 48, she said: 'I had been taking antidepressants, and after about 18 months, realised they were doing no good at all. I had terrible headaches and was told that my main problem was the menopause.

'I was also short of thyroid. Since taking Alexander lessons, I am still short of thyroid, but I haven't had any adverse symptoms. I am now able to breathe properly, and release all the tension in my neck and back.'

Good posture – the Alexander way

For an Alexander teacher, there is no fixed set of rules which constitutes good posture. It is not so much a correct way of standing or sitting, but of achieving the right balance. When we have good posture, we are relaxed, not stiff, and ready for action. We are not in a state of continual tension. To be ready and alert is not the same as being tense, strained and jumpy. Hunched shoulders are an obvious sign of bad posture, as are rounded backs.

Good posture is the body stance which allows balanced body alignment and makes for minimum expenditure of body energy. It is about conserving rather than wasting resources. In *Total Back Care* Christopher Hayne writes:

> *In order to regain our natural birthright and be able to live in an unrestrained natural manner, without any tension or pain, we have to learn how to listen to what our bodies are telling us. The way to postural health is through knowledge, awareness and graded activity.*

He goes on to say that each body type – ectomorphs, mesomorphs and endomorphs – has different postural tendencies. The tall, thin ectomorph will tend towards a slouched position, hunching shoulders, while the naturally short and stout endomorph will tend towards a bottom-heavy posture which puts extra strain on the lower back. The luckiest people are the middle of the road mesomorphs, who tend naturally to better balance. Alexander teachers will sum up the body shape and natural tendencies before suggesting any adjustments.

As posture tends to be a reflex action, which activates pathways within the central nervous system automatically, it is not easy to make alterations once the pathways have been established. Alexander believed that the pathways were usually established within the first four years of life, and thereafter became more or less automatic.

Usually, people only ever think about reprogramming themselves if, for some reason, their backs have been put out of action. Christopher Hayne thinks that such people are lucky, as they are motivated to relearn balance and realignment. But Alexander pupils do not have to wait for something to go wrong. It is not an exaggeration to say that, nowadays, just about everybody has developed wrong posture – and has to learn to change their reflexes before good posture can be learned.

In his book, *Total Back Care*, Christopher Hayne has this to say about the Alexander Technique:

> *Its postural and philosophical principles have enabled many back sufferers not only to become free of pain, but to learn to control their body posture and function in every situation . . . The Alexander Technique views the body and mind as a total psycho-physical organism and considers that the conscious mind can change the subconscious patterns of muscular usage. The key to the new body awareness advocated by Alexander is proper head and neck alignment as an initiator of total balanced posture . . . Your teacher will help you to experience a balanced relaxed posture, and to relate this to achieving 'normal function' in your daily activities. As the old harmful and stress-filled habits are replaced by the new balanced postural techniques, it is likely that you will gain an enhanced postural sense and feeling of control over yourself, a greater freedom from strain, as well as increased vigour.*

Back pain of one kind and another is by no means the only condition which can be eased, or possibly completely cured, by the Alexander Technique. Other chronic conditions which can be helped include:

- Rheumatism and arthritis

- Asthma

- Allergies

- Strokes

- Sports injuries

- Depression

- Migraine

- Gynaecological problems

- Breathing difficulties

- Stammering

- Addictions

Rheumatism

This condition, eventually suffered by about 80 per cent of the population, is any muscular ache or cramp. It begins with faulty distribution of body weight and builds up over a number of years until the joints become permanently wrongly positioned. Rheumatism and arthritis are joint problems which we can all expect sooner or later unless we learn to use our bodies correctly. However, they are not inevitable consequences of the ageing process, but conditions we bring on ourselves through chronic misuse.

Rheumatic-type conditions which can be greatly eased by Alexander lessons include leg cramps and what are often termed 'growing pains' in children. In fact, these are not growing pains at all; they are not caused by the growing process, but are brought about by strain, fatigue, or even such things as school phobia, a common problem which sets in when school has become a hateful place and the fears have grown to such an extent that the child will no longer attend. Emotional phobias are accompanied always by hunched, fearful postures, habitual tension manifesting itself in stammering, twitching or involuntary facial movements. All these can be cured by Alexander lessons. Even the phobia itself can be helped to go away.

Any child who complains of aches and pains in the arms and legs – particularly the legs – could benefit from Alexander lessons. They can easily be learned by youngsters.

Case history – Lilian Carpenter

A yoga teacher now in her sixties, Lilian Carpenter had cause to bless the Alexander Technique very early in life. As a child, she suffered a lot from rheumatism and is convinced that, but for Alexander lessons, she would not now be able to walk. As it is, she is far more upright and energetic than most people of her age.

She says: 'From experience, I believe that this Technique is by far the best kind of alternative therapy I have ever encountered. You are taught to give yourself orders to widen and broaden the back and release the neck. Once you can do this, you can feel the tension floating out. Above all, Alexander gives us an understanding of our physical make up, and knowledge of where we may be going wrong.

'I found that going for Alexander lessons was nothing short of pure bliss. The Technique seems to release something in the mind which links with the body, and then creates a two-way relationship which many people were unaware of before.'

Other aches and pains

Any muscular or joint ache at all will respond to Alexander lessons. In particular, the cracking and clicking of joints can be encouraged to go away. These clicks and snapping noises, often produced by those considered to be double jointed, put extra unnecessary strain on joints and eventually can lead to lack of mobility.

Very often, people in their thirties and forties notice their joints creaking. Though this does not necessarily mean they will eventually suffer arthritis, the clicks should not be ignored. They can be quite serious, and are indicative of wrong balance and lack of alignment.

Tennis elbow

Those conditions called 'tennis elbow' or 'frozen shoulder' are caused by small tears on the local muscles and can be extremely painful. The usual medical advice is to rest and take an aspirin, but the same kind of use is liable to result in an identical condition developing again. Alexander lessons can teach people how to prevent the build-up of strain which leads to frozen and painful joints and muscles.

Case history – Wilfred Murray

Wilfred Murray, a professional pianist, went for Alexander lessons after he suffered frozen shoulder, and was no longer able to play. He said: 'I first noticed problems about 15 years ago, but took no notice until one day I woke to find that my right arm was frozen. This is an occupational hazard for pianists, particularly with the right hand, as this is the one that does most of the work.

'I first went to my GP who diagnosed inflammation, but said there was nothing he could do to help. He simply recommended rest. An osteopath I visited couldn't help either.

'Then I got to hear about Alexander lessons. I discovered that my complaint was actually tendonitis, a condition very similar to tennis elbow.

'The teacher showed me a different, more relaxed way of practising, one which caused less tension on muscles and joints. When I started doing Alexander lessons, I discovered that my playing actually improved with less practice. Not that these lessons are a substitute for practice, but most professional musicians over-practice, not always realising that they are not necessarily improving.'

Wilfred Murray found that unlearning bad habits did adversely affect his playing for a time. 'But after I learned the technique it seemed as if my playing began to improve with less effort than before. Since going for Alexander lessons I have never had a frozen arm, but know that the trouble could always come back again. I know now how to look out for the signs.'

Breathing problems and asthma

These are also caused by wrong use of the body, and in particular, wrong 'primary control'.

Case history – Fiona Ross

A librarian from Scotland, she had suffered from chronic asthma since she was a small child, and it had left her with a permanently bent back which no exercises seemed to help. When she first heard about the Alexander Technique, she wondered if this might help.

She said: 'My asthma had really messed up my life. It had stopped me getting a decent education or having a social life, and I'm certain it affected my personality.

'I had always been very self-conscious about my crooked back, and would never go swimming, for example, because I hated the way I looked in a swimming costume. I felt that all eyes were on me.

'The first thing that surprised me about my Alexander teacher was that she didn't want to know anything about my history of ill health. Before I went, I heard that the teacher touched you, and this worried me rather a lot.

'But after the initial lesson, I knew it was the right therapy for me at last.' After three years of lessons, Fiona's asthma is completely under control, and her back has become straight.

'I never thought this was possible,' she said, 'I simply never get attacks of asthma as I used to. I know that it isn't actually cured, and if I stop practising the Alexander Technique it is liable to come back. But nowadays, I never have to take time off work, whereas previously I was sometimes off for a month.

'Everybody has commented on my changed appearance – it is quite dramatic. An added bonus is that I have lost a lot of weight, even though I didn't diet, or particularly try to slim.'

The asthmatic, says Wilfred Barlow, has to be taught how to stop wrong ways of breathing, as it is mainly this which has caused the trouble in the first place. Ordinary breathing exercises do not help the asthmatic very much and in fact studies on the subject have indicated that after these exercises many asthmatics breathe even less efficiently than before.

The asthmatic, explained Barlow, does not need breathing exercises, but rather, breathing *education*. He writes:

> *He needs a minute analysis of his faulty breathing habits and clear instruction on how to replace them by an improved use of his chest. Such chest-use cannot be separated out from a consideration of the general manner of use.*

Of course, as all Alexander teachers point out, the physical problems can never be separated from emotional or personality considerations. Wilfred Barlow considers that all asthmatics and sufferers from bronchitis have personality problems, and that the two go together. Many back doctors now believe that chronic back sufferers carry mental burdens on their backs for years, in much the same way as Christian in John Bunyan's *Pilgrim's Progress*.

At the same time as helping pupils to relieve the physical problems, the Alexander teacher will try to discover the mental and emotional tensions which accompany the physical pain. These will be considered in greater detail in the following chapter.

4

The emotional
benefits

One of the most important teachings of the Alexander Technique is that body, mind and emotions cannot be separated from one another. Whatever affects the body will immediately be transmitted to the mind, and vice versa.

We are now quite used to this concept, with the emergence of interest in holistic medicine, which treats the individual as a functioning whole, rather than a machine whose individual parts may have gone wrong. When Alexander first formulated the concept, though, he was many decades ahead of his time, although he knew nothing of the science of biochemistry which is now studied so minutely. Investigations by modern scientists have shown that the mind and body are indeed affected by each other, as they are interconnected by hormones, neurotransmitters, enzymes and other chemical messengers.

Mental stress

The network of biochemical interactions is so complicated that even now we do not understand it fully, but it is now generally accepted by most doctors that mental stress can result in bodily illness. To give an example, when we are emotionally overstressed, this causes overproduction of the chemical adrenaline, which affects the workings of the heart, circulation and other vital organs.

In order to reduce the amount of mental stress we feel, we

may start drinking alcohol or taking legal or illegal drugs. Unfortunately, none of these substances ever right the stress, but simply damp down our perception of it. In time, they also affect the workings of the nerves, joints, muscles and bones. The net result is that we get ever more ill, and the body gets ever more stressed.

The trouble is, it is difficult to work on the mind alone. Over the past 20 years or so, scientists have developed very strong psychotropic drugs, which actually alter perceptions in the brain. They may also have the effect of destroying the immune system, increasing susceptibility to infections and diseases such as cancer, rheumatism and arthritis. But these drugs do not and cannot actually cure our problems – they just damp down our mental anguish and unease. Underneath, it is still there.

Alexander understood that the purely psychiatric approach was not enough. If you work on the mind alone, without paying attention to the body, there is a distinct danger that the problem will only be masked, rather than cured. Those who are mentally and emotionally troubled often show this in their body language. They walk with hunched shoulders, have nervous twitches, develop self-effacing mannerisms, or stoop and allow their heads to slump on to their necks. Whenever people experience anguish, they show this in their physical stance – putting their head in their hands, twisting themselves into agonising postures, looking sad, angry or bewildered and unbelieving. There are always intense physical reactions to mental stress. Some of these we can help; others, such as increased production of adrenaline and other stress hormones, may become involuntary after a time.

But by working on the body, these mental strains can be allowed to come to the surface and evaporate. When posture and 'primary control' are kept correct, it becomes much more difficult for emotional stress to enter the body, and to stay there. Whenever we hunch our shoulders, or walk with a stoop, we are showing the rest of the world that we are troubled – and our bodies respond by becoming inharmonious and troubled themselves. Disease and illnesses of all kinds are nothing more than manifestations of a lack of harmony in the human system.

There seems little doubt that the amount of stress we suffer is increasing all the time. Medical science has been very successful in helping to eradicate the big killer diseases of the past, such as smallpox and plagues. Public health measures have also ensured that (in the West at least) we are no longer in danger of contracting cholera, typhoid, or other conditions which come from a polluted water supply, bad housing, or unhygienic practices.

The problem of mental stress, leading to such physical ills as cancer, rheumatism and arthritis – even the most traditionally-minded doctors now allow that mental disturbance can lead to chronic physical conditions – seems to be, at the moment, intractable. The sheer number of prescriptions written each year for tranquillisers and sleeping pills, as well as the amount of alcohol drunk, indicates how huge the problem is.

Learning the Alexander Technique is a very potent tool for driving out long-held stresses from the system. It is a bodily, postural technique which has profound mental implications. Studies on sport and exercise have shown that physical exercise really can help to reduce stress levels in the brain. It does this mainly by encouraging the release of endorphins, the body's natural painkillers, which enable us to overcome stress. The trouble is, we may have been misusing our bodies for so many years that ordinary exercises can no longer put them right. This is one of the main reasons for the proliferation of sports injuries, and also the incidences of joggers suffering from heart attacks, or, less seriously, incapacitating knee and joint problems.

The fact is, most of us don't know how to use our bodies. We have lost the art, and therein lies the inherent danger of formerly sedentary people taking up sudden exercise. Taking up running, squash or tennis in later life cannot undo the postural wrongs of a lifetime. An added danger is that there is only temporary removal of stress, anyway. Runners commonly experience the 'runner's high' – the good feeling which makes them continue to jog each morning. But once the high goes down, there is likely to be depression. In this way, running, or any other highly active sport, can become an addiction, a way of trying to attain the sought-after high.

With the Alexander Technique, there are no swings of high and low, as the idea is to enable permanent changes to take place, changes which mean that the vicious cycle of the interaction of bodily and mental stress is broken for ever. Once the technique is learned and understood, bodily harmony will result. This will mean not only better functioning, but also a calmer, more relaxed and better-balanced human being.

Breathing problems and the emotional connection

All those who are under undue stress will be breathing wrongly. Alexander stated this as a fact over 50 years ago, and it has been confirmed by doctors specialising in heart and circulatory problems. Whenever fear and panic set in, breathing patterns alter. We can all experience this for ourselves at moments of actual fear, or when experiencing it vicariously, such as when watching a horror film. We can observe sweaty palms, heightened heartbeat and increased pulse. Many people, though, feel fear not just occasionally but all the time. They are always nervous, always afraid, always panicky. This very nervousness can become a habit, and is quickly translated to the body, so that shallow or panic breathing can become a reflex action and therefore habitual and unconscious. Wrong breathing further has the effect of altering body functions by changing the amount of oxygen and carbon dioxide which should be in the body.

We all know that the way we breathe is intimately connected with emotional states. When we are calm and at peace, breathing becomes deep, regular and relaxed. The pulse rate slows down, and all bodily functions are in harmony. When we are excited or troubled, the first thing to alter is the way we breathe. At times of increased stress, we tend to overbreathe, in quick, chest-heaving pants; this is technically known as **hyperventilation**. What happens is that shallow breathing takes place only in the upper part of the chest, so the balance of carbon dioxide and oxygen are altered and far too much carbon dioxide is expelled from the body.

When this becomes the habitual way of breathing, in time every organ in the body is affected, and can cause a variety of symptoms. Overbreathing is a normal response to excitement or danger. It allows the body to take in additional oxygen to prepare it for quick action, if needed. Most people, for example, will overbreathe if they run for a bus. When the body is not keyed up for extra action, the breathing should become calmer and deeper.

The condition of overbreathing can be extremely serious if untreated. Fluctuating levels of carbon dioxide have the immediate effect of making people breathless, weak and tired. This sensitises nerve endings to such an extent that in the end, any kind of normal life may become impossible. In severe cases, any form of touch can become unbearable, even that from a loved one. Alexander teachers often find that their pupils initially cannot bear to be touched and shrink away from the most gentle pressure. These are usually people who have been overbreathing for many years.

Habitual hyperventilators may also be abnormally sensitive to noise, petrol fumes, perfume, wool, pollen, house dust or certain foods.

The trouble is, doctors do not always recognise hyperventilation, and may treat the condition, or the variety of symptoms, with sleeping pills, tranquillisers or beta-blockers, all of which mess up the body's natural workings even more.

The classic sign of a hyperventilator is frequent pins and needles. Most of the work on the condition has been carried out in Britain by Dr Claude Lum, until recently a chest physician at the famous Papworth Hospital near Cambridge. While working on heart patients, he discovered that the all-important flow of blood to the brain is controlled by the amount of carbon dioxide the blood contains. When the CO_2 pressure is too low, blood vessels in the brain contract, and the circulatory flow is reduced. Symptoms of the condition are:

- Sudden changes of behaviour

- Nervousness

- Inability to concentrate

- Headaches

- Tiredness

Almost all of Alexander's own patients were suffering from the above symptoms.

Athletes, singers and actors are particularly prone to hyperventilation, as their careers mean they have to breathe in certain ways. Men and women can suffer equally, and the condition has its roots in stress. The typical male hyperventilator is a harassed executive who has work problems, and finds it difficult to unwind when off duty. The upright, military, stiff upper lip kind of man is a prime candidate for this condition. In order to maintain his military stance, he may well overbreathe continually.

Hyperventilators are often particular personality types. They are usually highly active, talented people who are perfectionists. For some reason, stress has taken hold of their lives and they are no longer able to relax and let it go.

The cure for this condition is to learn to breathe properly. It will be remembered that Alexander first stumbled on his technique when he suffered from voice problems, caused by an inability to breathe properly when he threw his head back (see Chapter 1). He therefore concentrated greatly on helping people to ease their sufferings through correct breathing. Through proper breathing education, patients can be helped to let go of their stress, not allowing it to build up in the body through wrong breathing patterns, and so develop into full-scale illness.

The recent popularity of yoga and meditation has grown up mainly in response to the problem of overbreathing which, eventually, stops people from living full lives. But usually, these techniques are not specifically tailored to the individual. Although people may feel calmer when they meditate, their bodies may not be helped to realign. Also, physical yoga may not have the desired effect, as it is an Eastern practice for which Western bodies are not always well adapted.

Alexander teachers are required to have a detailed knowledge of anatomy and physiology and how to right ingrained bodily wrongs. Only the Alexander method can work to release the pent-up emotions and stresses which have led to the chronic overbreathing problem – something which, once established, can never be altered by willpower alone, or even simple breathing exercises.

Fiona Ross, the asthmatic who gained so much benefit from learning the Alexander Technique (see page 50), soon came to realise that there was a strong emotional component to her problems. She said: 'One of the things that troubled me at first was that I was just not prepared for my strong emotional reaction to the Alexander lessons. They are very gentle, so you don't expect it. Once I reacted really violently, and had a seizure. It seemed to me then that the sessions had awakened some awful, long-repressed emotions, and all I could do was to shake and shake.

'I felt that everything inside me, in fact my whole life, was being shaken up dramatically and I was being forced to rethink everything. I had to ask myself why I was doing what I was doing, and how I could go forward.

'No treatments I had had in the past sparked off this kind of reaction,' she continued. 'But I knew somehow that all the things which were coming out had to come out, if I was to get better. My emotions and the asthma were so intimately linked, I could not really separate them from each other. But that is what other doctors had tried to do.'

Other stress-related complaints

These are mainly what alternative health expert Brian Inglis has termed 'The diseases of civilisation'. They include:

- Cancer

- Heart and circulatory problems

- Rheumatism and arthritis

- Depression

- Migraine

- Undue tiredness

- Muscle fatigue

- Insomnia

- Skin problems

- Susceptibility to infections

One of the most obviously stress-related illnesses is **hypertension**, or dangerously raised blood pressure. There are drugs one can take to lessen high blood pressure, but these cannot cure the condition, or pinpoint the underlying cause of the disease.

It is now accepted by most doctors, that emotional factors are high on the list of precipitatory causes of high blood pressure. Some doctors have implicated salt content in the diet as a cause, but as heart and stress expert Dr Malcolm Carruthers has pointed out, 'It's not so much what you're eating as what's eating you.' Emotions have a very strong effect on the heart and circulatory systems.

A high-pressure job often means, literally, just that. People who feel in their heads that they are under pressure, will instantly translate this to their bodies via the heart and circulation. Fear works to raise blood pressure and keep it high. Many people live in a state of constant fear these days. They are worried that they may lose their jobs, that they may not be able to establish good personal relationships, that they may lose their spouse, that their children may not be a credit, that the house will fall down, that the world will blow itself up. Often worry in itself becomes a habit.

The trouble is, the heart – which pumps harder when there is an emergency – does not distinguish between a genuine emergency, and one which remains in the mind. Worry can send blood pressure soaring just as high as if there was an actual disaster.

Alexander teachers are often able to bring blood pressure down considerably just by working on the muscles. In his book, *The Alexander Principle*, Wilfred Barlow states:

I have found blood pressure to drop by as much as 30 points after a half-hour re-educational session in which tense muscles were relaxed: and it seems reasonable to suggest that since most blood vessels traverse or are surrounded by muscles, any over-contraction of the muscle is bound to squeeze the lumen (cavity) of the blood vessel and thereby make it more difficult for the blood to be pumped through them by the heart. The less the obstruction to the blood flow, the less the pressure.

Other stress-related problems which can be helped by an understanding of the Alexander Technique are:

● Gastro-intestinal troubles

● Ulcers of all kinds

● Anorexia nervosa

Eating problems are very often related to stress initially – and then a reaction is set up in the body whereby digestion becomes difficult, taste buds are blunted, mechanism of body cells alter, and the whole digestive system goes out of balance. Wilfred Barlow also says that undiagnosed pain in the stomach – a very common cause of admission to hospital, especially in men – is very often caused by allowing stress to build up. Emotional stress can easily be held in the stomach, as most of us have experienced. Whenever we are nervous or frightened, we commonly say we feel sick 'to the pit of our stomach', or that our stomach 'turned over'. People with chronic stomach problems, says Barlow, often have ingrained postural imbalance. In fact, the two almost always go together. In his book he writes:

More often than not, these patients will be found to have a slight sideways displacement of the thorax on the lower back and often a rotary twist of the dorso-lumbar spine with associated muscle spasm. This should always be looked for in cases of unexplained abdominal discomfort.

Wilfred Barlow also says that the Alexander Technique can successfully treat migraine sufferers, epileptics and those suffering from gynaecological problems. All these diseases have emotional components, and all will eventually cause bodily misuse. Alexander had particular success with neuralgia and all types of facial pain and spasms.

Accident-proneness, or habitual clumsiness, is another condition whcih can be treated successfully by Alexander methods. Again, there is a strong emotional component in being accident-prone, as habitually clumsy people are those who have become graceless and unco-ordinated through lack of self-esteem and self-confidence.

Over exertion

It is common, in our society, for us to put far too much effort into tasks. This tendency very much interested Alexander, as he considered that it was one of the prime factors in developing wrong body use. The question is: *why* are we so prone to over-exertion? One explanation is imitation. As small children, we imitate those around us, and if these people put too much effort into everything, then we will too – simply because that is what we see as normal.

But over and above that, is the fact that many of us today are engaged on tasks which do not please us. This sets in very early at school, when we are asked to perform activities we may hate. Whenever a person hates or resents the task in hand, it is likely to be executed with far too much effort. As well as the muscular effort needed for the job, there will also be large amounts of anger experienced. Anger and resentment always have immediate physical outlets. The facial expression will change, and as facial muscles and nerve endings connect up to others in the brain and down the spine, the anger will be translated to the muscles.

Small children often carry out orders from adults with what we normally term 'bad grace'. Whenever this happens, there will be unco-ordinated body movements and postural imbalances. As we get older, the number of distasteful tasks we are required to do, or feel we must do, seems to grow and grow. Most housewives hate housework, so they will do this inwardly seething, but at the same time feeling huge amounts of guilt. Anything done out of a sense of duty rather than because one enjoys the task, is likely to be accompanied by unnecessarily excessive physical effort.

Housework seems tiring, even though most homes are now equipped with gadgets that are supposed to make the job easier. We buy vacuum cleaners, dishwashers, washing machines and so on in order to save physical effort, and have more energy left over for other tasks, yet most people frenetically load or push round their machines, thus doubling the effort really needed, simply because they hate the task.

There is no obvious way to learn to love housework, gardening, driving, or any other everyday activity which may be resented. What the Alexander Technique can do, though, is to teach people to put appropriate amounts of effort in, so that there is no residual stress or resentment when the task is complete. Hate and anger build up inside the system and have a cumulative effect, so that each new bout of housework or gardening (or whatever) seems more hateful than the last.

When embarking on distasteful tasks, it is helpful to remember Alexander's instruction to release the neck, widen and broaden the back (described in detail in the following chapter) and concentrate on these, rather than the task in hand. This will make time pass more quickly and allow such jobs to have a positive side.

Types A and B

The Alexander method recognises that we are all individuals, and have different problems and solutions. This is why the lessons are almost always carried out on a one-to-one basis, as what suits one person may be quite wrong for another.

In particular, practitioners of the technique understand the distinction between Type A and Type B people, a distinction first formulated by American doctors Meher Friedman and Ray Rosenman in their book *Type A Behaviour and Your Heart*. Type As are high-achievers, people who are always impatient, who tend to do everything, including eating and drinking, very quickly. Type B people, by contrast, are those who are relaxed and calm about what they do, feel no need to hurry and are not continually preoccupied with feelings of frustration, anger and impatience.

Type A people are, in Alexander terms, the most obvious 'endgainers', in such a hurry to reach their goal that they hardly ever pause to consider the 'means whereby'. Alexander himself started out as a typical Type A, restless, ambitious, with a tendency to put people's backs up, always looking for new challenges, with a low threshold of boredom. He probably remained a Type A all his life, but formulation of his technique enabled him to temper this with correct use of the body.

Most Type A people misuse their bodies badly and suffer from backache, ulcers and head and neck problems, as well as a tendency towards developing heart trouble in middle age. These are people who normally never consider their bodies until something starts to go seriously wrong. They would probably view conscious relaxation as a waste of time, as it would seem like doing nothing. The thought of easing themselves gently into their chair with spine-lengthening, slow movements and getting up by imagining there is an invisible string pulling them skywards, would come very hard.

Type As tend to plonk themselves into a chair, slump over their work, rush around all day long and drive cars with unnecessary ferocity. They also find it hard to listen to what others are saying, and interrupt or finish sentences for people. They are often clever enough to conceal the fact that they can't listen to others, and learn such conversational gambits as, 'How interesting', and 'Oh really', giving the illusion of listening, when their minds are in reality racing ahead, following their own trains of thought.

Meyer and Rosenman contended that Type A behaviour, if allowed to carry on unchecked over a long period, would predispose to heart disease and serious circulatory problems. The main characteristic of Type A behaviour, they said, was a kind of restless, impatient striving. Type A people are always setting themselves targets, trying to get things done in an ever-shorter time.

Type Bs, by contrast, are unhurried and unharried, but this does not mean they are not successful. In fact, it is possible to be more successful as a Type B, because there is not the same risk of running yourself into the ground by unnecessary hurry.

The main problem with Type A behaviour is that sufferers in the end cannot choose *not* to hurry and rush everywhere. They become restless and impatient in their everyday behaviour, and simply cannot take it easy, even if they have been advised by their doctor that they should try and relax. Type As simply can't relax.

As most cannot change their behaviour by an act of will, Alexander lessons are ideal, as they teach a completely new way of going about everyday life. The great majority of Alexander's own pupils were Type As – aggressive, striving, and anxious. It is the anxiety which makes them hurry all the time, even when there is no need.

Another major problem with Type A people is that eventually they lose their power of thought and reflection. For true creativity to take place, the brain has to go into 'alpha' rhythms – the slower rates associated with daydreaming. Type A people spend most of their lives at 'beta' – the conscious waking rhythm associated with carrying out logical, routine tasks. During Alexander lessons, the mind is helped to go into the alpha rhythm, the calm, relaxed brain wave. Dr David Lewis, author of *The Alpha Plan*, which teaches tense, anxious people how to relax and arrive at the alpha brainwave, writes:

> *Alpha is generally associated with feelings of relaxed awareness. The mind is tranquil yet receptive. These brain waves are also associated with pleasurable and rewarding activities.*

Alpha and beta brain waves are not airy-fairy nonsense, but actualities which can easily be measured on an EEG (electroencephalograph) machine. Alpha waves have a frequency of around 8 and 14 cycles per second.

The beta waves: frequency 15–22 cycles per second, are associated with active thinking, paying attention, concentrating, paying attention to the outside world and solving problems. The two other types of brain waves, usually known as delta and theta, are associated with sleep. During very deep sleep, delta waves, with a frequency of 0.5 to 4 cycles per second, are the only ones in operation.

Small children, says David Lewis, produce delta and theta waves frequently. As we grow up, alpha starts to take over, until by the time we are adult, we spend most of our waking hours at beta. The ability to get into the alpha rhythm means that the brain is freed from niggling worries, and is helped to free itself from negative emotions.

During Alexander's time, it was not possible to measure brain waves electrically. But the advent of the EEG machine, and our subsequent knowledge about brain waves, is yet another indication of how far ahead of his time Alexander was – and how right in so many ways. He knew that great thinkers like Aldous Huxley had to allow themselves to go into alpha if creativity was to continue – which is why Alexander suggested taking a walk or having a relaxation break every one-and-a-half hours.

The standard Alexander lying-down practice – which pupils are asked to do every day, and which is described in detail in the following chapter – helps the brain to go into alpha. This aids future concentration and creativity and breaks the cycle of anxious, negative thoughts.

Performance anxiety

The vast majority of Alexander's original pupils were professional performers – actors, musicians, singers – who felt they needed to improve their technique, or who had got stuck during rehearsals and couldn't seem to improve.

All of us suffer to some extent from performance anxiety, and one way to decrease this is to take drugs known as beta-blockers. These put a kind of straitjacket round the heart, and stop tremble and the palpitations associated with having to give any kind of public performance. Until recently, it was very common for snooker players to rely on beta blockers – but these have now been banned from top-flight competitions unless it can be proved that the player actually needs them for medical reasons.

Beta blockers do not take away the anxiety – but they stop manifestations of it. It has been shown in tests at the Royal Free Hospital in North London that violinists – who particularly need steady hands – actually performed better with beta blockers than without.

The trouble with beta-blockers, as with all drugs, is that they have both welcome and unwelcome side effects. In men, beta-blockers increase the risk of developing impotence, and they can also cause feelings of nausea, vomiting, fatigue and dizziness. According to Dr Arabella Melville and Colin Johnson, authors of *Cured to Death – The Effects of Prescription Drugs*, beta-blockers are also associated with various blood disorders and occasionally severe conditions such as congestive heart failure and heart block. As they cause slowing of the heart, low blood pressure and cold extremities, they can also lead to Reynaud's Disease, where blood supply to fingers and toes is cut off. They can also cause depression, sleep and vision disturbances and skin rashes.

Numerous studies have shown that beta-blockers do reduce hypertension and bring down blood pressure to more normal levels. The Alexander Technique can, however, act as a natural beta-blocker without any of the adverse side effects of this prescription drug.

Case history – Paul Collins

The Technique can also help to remove the 'block' suffered by many performers. Paul Collins is a professional violinist who decided to train as an Alexander teacher after he found the technique made all the difference to his playing.

He said: 'When I was about 40, I began having severe problems with my playing. Like most string players, I had been experiencing muscular problems for some time and although I heard the alarm bells ringing, I couldn't seem to do anything to reduce the tension.

'Over the years, of course, I had become very unbalanced and stressed on one side. The problem was, how to get my muscles back into their proper shape. I eventually managed to do this by an understanding of the primary control.

'Like most musicians, I had been for medical advice and nobody was able to help me. But the Alexander lessons changed my whole outlook, and my playing. Although you work only on the body, the technique deeply affects the mind. A lot of the stresses that musicians feel in their muscles are caused by anxiety and mental tension – you have to keep performing, and are anxious about being good enough, and being able to play well. This anxiety in itself causes muscular tension to remain in the system.

'Coupled with the hours of practice all professional musicians have to do each day, this means that after 20 years or so you are likely to be in a very bad way indeed. I found I had to give up the violin completely for three months, in order to enable my body to regain its alignment.

'When you are well co-ordinated physically, there is a good feedback between mind and body. Most of my pupils now, whether they are musicians or not, are under enormous stress, and that is one main reason why their bodies are out of alignment.'

Pianist Wilfred Murray also found that the Alexander Technique was the only therapy that could help him. He said: 'Alexander himself understood that very often, when professional performers imagine they are practising, or rehearsing, when in fact, what they are doing is increasing the stress and not gaining anything. If you don't practise in the right way, or with the right attitude, you can actually lose something, and ingrain bad mental and physical habits.

'You practise and practise, trying to get a piece right, but you are always in danger of becoming mechanical and losing some of the magic and spontaneity. When I began learning the Technique, I found that I could actually improve with less practice – as my concentration was greater, and my stress levels reduced.

'What it really comes down to is learning to practise with a different attitude. As you become more relaxed, you can let things come through. You learn that there is a limit to what you can consciously arrange with your mind. You also discover that not all of the practice need be at the piano. You can think about what you are doing, reflect on the music and how you are going to interpret it. The Technique seems to free some blockage in the mind – a blockage that all performers feel at times.

'I also found that Alexander lessons brought out more of my own personality, so that I could put more of myself into the playing and give less mechanical renderings. But apart from the greatly improved playing, I also have a greater sense of general wellbeing and health.'

He said that one huge problem with performers of all kinds is that they get so far and then seem to hit a brick wall. After that, however much they practise or rehearse, they never seem to get better. 'At this stage,' said Wilfred Murray, 'they may decide to give up their careers for good. The more they practise, the more stressed they seem to become, and the more likely they are to lose what they have already gained. For these people, a knowledge of the Alexander Technique could help them get over the mental block which is impeding their progress. It's their attitude which needs to change. Unless they can be helped to overcome the stress, despair can set in. Of course, the Alexander Technique is not going to turn every pianist into a Horovitz, every ballerina into an Alicia Markova. It's not a substitute for native talent. But it could save very many promising performers from giving up their careers when they hit a hard patch, and never seem to progress.'

Wilfred Murray added that a potent benefit was that he was now much better tempered. Stress and anxiety of all kinds tend to make people bad-tempered. One characteristic of Type A people is that they often become very bad-tempered in middle age, and are like this almost all the time. For them, bad temper becomes a normal way of reacting to situations.

Detecting mental states

Wilfred Barlow, who spent ten years working with Alexander, says that over a period of time he was able to observe that FM's approach provided a way of detecting mental states which no other therapy could diagnose so readily. Anxiety was always accompanied by acute muscle tension, and the connection between negative mental states and physical misuse was always very close indeed.

Barlow discovered over the years that arm tension was always associated with hostility, and buttock and thigh tension with sexual problems. Those plagued by persistent headaches also suffered from chronic strain, anxiety and apprehension. Writer's cramp – now usually known as repetitive strain injury – often occurs when there is unconcious anger in the mind of the writer. This manifests itself first in clenching of the forearm and then to unnatural head and neck postures to counteract this.

'In many other ways,' Barlow writes, 'it became clear that

the mentally sick were physically tense.' He adds that it is actually impossible to separate the physical and the psychological. Of course, one does not have to be suffering from a diagnosable mental illness to be suffering from tension and anxiety: these states are experienced by everybody today. Electrical methods of recording muscle tension have now largely confirmed everything Alexander had to say on the subject.

All mental states, whether positive or negative, are accompanied by physical movements of one kind or another. These may be very slight, such as increased blinking, or extremely noticeable, as with hyperactive children. Tension states always occur when there is emotional strain. It is only by learning proper use of the muscles that we can prevent negative feedback. Correct use of the muscles enables more positive feedback to be given to the mind, so that both mind and body can be freed from habitual tension.

Most of all, the Alexander Technique aids people to free themselves from the prison of their past, so that former negative attitudes do not blight the future. It enables pupils to let go of the fear and stress which may have stopped them from enjoying life to the full.

It achieves this in the most stress-free way possible – by gentle redirection of muscular activity. The next chapter will describe just what happens during a typical course of Alexander lessons.

5

The Alexander course of lessons

Anybody who wants to gain maximum benefit from the Alexander Technique should ideally fix up a course of lessons from a qualified teacher. New pupils will soon discover that these lessons are like no other kind of therapy.

They are not quite a series of exercises, they are not merely relaxation or a set of postures, as in yoga – rather, they encompass all three disciplines. Though they seem gentle, they are actually very hard work, as you learn to allow your body to move in different ways, to shed old, bad habits and substitute new ways of conducting yourself. Learning and ingraining the new habits can be quite a struggle.

The students

Most people who book up Alexander lessons have suffered bad back problems, chronic migraine, or a joint condition such as arthritis. They are very often people who have 'tried everything', who have already consulted their doctor, and specialists, only to find that their problem worsens. In many cases, Alexander lessons come at the end of the line of a long search for a cure, or at least alleviation of the condition.

The other main group of people who may consult an Alexander teacher are professional performers – singers, actors, musicians, for example – who have somehow got stuck, and are having problems in progressing. As we saw in the last chapter, violinists consult Alexander specialists when they suffer from repetitive strain injuries, and pianists when they find their practice seems to be becoming counterproductive. The Alexander Technique has always been popular with those practising the performing arts, and several music colleges offer Alexander lessons.

But you don't have to have anything wrong with you to benefit from a course of lessons. Most of us are using our bodies in wrong or inefficient ways and storing up muscular troubles for later life. Also, it is likely that we are holding ancient stresses, anxieties, grudges and negativities in our bodies.

It is not an exaggeration to say that Alexander lessons can help everybody, whatever their age, sex or bodily condition.

What to expect

Alexander lessons are enjoyable, and contain none of the off-putting requirements of, say, a typical exercise or yoga class. For one thing, you do not have to wear special clothes. You can have lessons in whatever you happen to be wearing, although loose tracksuits are recommended.

As the lessons are on a one-to-one basis, there is no competitive aspect, as can happen in an exercise class. You don't have to worry about what the others are doing, feeling embarrassed because you can't do the tricks. There is no prancing about, and there are no bodily contortions to achieve.

Nor will the teacher ask you awkward or difficult questions about your parents, your childhood, your relationships. Alexander teachers are taught to observe strains and tensions in bodily movements; they do not need to probe in a psycho-analytic way. Nor will teachers tell you what terrible shape your body is in. They will just gently guide you to better ways of being, and enable you to establish primary control.

Alexander lessons are not usually available on the National Health, although they may be allowed by private insurance schemes, if recommended by a doctor, or if a qualified doctor is also an Alexander teacher. The number of lessons each person needs varies, depending on what is wrong, but 20 is an average amount. This is the length of time it takes most people to re-establish good bodily habits, and to learn and assimilate the Technique.

A first lesson

Elizabeth Atkinson qualified as an Alexander teacher in 1976, and now gives lessons in her South London flat, and at Goldsmith's College, University of London. She also trains potential Alexander teachers. One of the rooms in her flat has been turned into an Alexander consulting room, and contains a long hard table and a chair – and very little else. She gives lessons wearing a tracksuit and advises her pupils to do the same. It is far easier, she says, to see how you move, and how your joints and muscles are aligned if you wear something loose and light, rather than a business suit or anything constricting.

As I myself went to Elizabeth for Alexander lessons, I shall describe how she conducts her courses. All Alexander teachers give lessons in slightly different ways, but the object is the same – to help the pupil undo wrong body usage, and learn better habits. The stages I describe were those she used for me, and will not necessarily be the same for all students, as the Alexander teacher's approach is to discover each individual's particular needs and work on them.

At the first lesson, she described briefly what the Alexander Technique is about, and explained that it is emphatically not a series of correct postures to be learned slavishly. 'After all,' she said, 'What good are yoga postures when you are sitting at your desk during the day?' The Alexander procedure is very much geared to each individual, and how each person relates to his or her body, and the world in general.

She began by asking questions to find out why I had come, and what my health problems might be. She also asked about any childhood accidents, or illnesses. Very often, a pupil will have had bad asthma as a child, and grown out of it and forgotten about it. But for an Alexander teacher, this information is important, as it will often give vital clues about bodily postures now, as an adult.

Elizabeth finds that at first, pupils often assert that there is nothing whatever wrong with them. 'When you probe a little deeper though,' she said, 'you may discover that they fell off a tree at nine, and were in plaster for several weeks, or laid up with scarlet or glandular fever. As Alexander teachers, we know that any physical or emotional trauma tends to get stored up, and remains in the system for many years. I often find, after a few lessons, that people will start wheezing, and I ask whether they ever had asthma. At first they may say no, then remember that they did.'

She will also want to know what surgical operations, if any, a pupil may have had. The reason for this is that, during Alexander lessons, old operation scars can suddenly start hurting again.

'I don't do a medical examination like a doctor,' she explained. 'And there is never any question of people lying on a table and taking their clothes off. But I can always feel by touching muscles and joints when something is not right.'

Elizabeth then asks pupils why they have come for lessons and what they hope to get out of them. At the initial consultation she explains just what the Technique can and cannot do. She tells people at the outset that the Alexander course is not a magic cure-all for every single disease, emotional problem or chronic condition.

Perhaps the most important aspect of the technique for people to understand is that Alexander teachers never concentrate on illnesses, or dwell on personal problems. That is not their concern. They always ask people to do things as if they were in full health and strength, and make no allowances for backache, migraine or whatever. This is the only way they can ascertain just what is wrong, by observing which actions the pupil is unable to perform or finds in any way difficult.

Elizabeth also explains the very difficult concept that some people actually need their illnesses and would be lost without them. This is very hard for many people to understand, as most of us cannot easily see any great benefit in being ill. But in the context of Alexander teaching, this becomes comprehensible. Above all, Alexander himself taught that we are creatures of habit and that we can get used to anything at all. In time, we actually get to like what we are used to, and cannot easily let go.

Perhaps this concept becomes easier to understand in terms

of giving up a habit such as smoking. Most smokers know perfectly well that cigarettes are bad for their health. Although some manage to give up, many say that they enjoy smoking, that it is one of the pleasures of their life, and that they cannot imagine not smoking. For these people, the habit has become so ingrained that it is almost part of them; the habit of smoking is hard to relinquish because it has become an addiction.

Exactly the same process can happen with illnesses. Nobody should ever imagine that illnesses are all bad. Very often, being a chronic invalid gives an individual a valid excuse not to do things they find distasteful. They can always plead a bad back, their nerves, their terrible headache, their arthritis – and people will understand. If these people became well again, they might have to take on more responsibility for themselves. While they are ill, though, they are assured of sympathy, concern and help from others. Chronically ill people also command attention from family, friends and doctors. This might be lost if they suddenly became well.

Not only that, over the years, they become attached to their illness, and the actual illness may be part of their 'personality'. Such people may have organised their lives around the illness. What would they do if this long-ingrained lifestyle were to be taken away from them?

An Alexander teacher has to find out at the first lesson what is the pupil's actual attitude to his or her own illness or condition, then to assess how, or whether, this person can be helped. No reputable teacher will take fees from people they cannot help. Teachers also have to establish whether there is a willingness to learn, as the technique requires great commitment and motivation from the pupil. Sometimes, people can't be bothered to learn new ways of moving. For this reason, teachers usually like to establish at the outset how the pupil has heard of the Technique, and what persuaded them to come. If they have been sent by a spouse or parent, very often there will not be the necessary motivation to take the maximum from the lessons.

As Elizabeth Atkinson takes a case history, she will assess all these factors. She wants to discover the pupil's attitude to himself or herself, and also to other people. She says: 'I am listening to the information, but all the time I am asking myself: is this person in a state of panic, or deep anxiety? As they talk, I will observe closely their body language, their gestures. Most people have no idea how much they give themselves away as they speak – and not only by what they say.'

At this point, the question of payment will come up. Most Alexander teachers will be very direct on the question of payment, as they feel this must be part of the commitment. Elizabeth says she is strict about paying fees on time, and makes people pay for missed appointments, if not enough advance notice is given. 'In the early days,' she explained, 'this was a problem area for many teachers, as they didn't like to ask for money. Now that proper training courses have been established, and being an Alexander teacher is a livelihood for many people, we can't afford to be lax. We also know that there is a big psychological component in paying for lessons.

'Most of us charge the minimum we can, but we understand that people do not value the lessons unless they are charged an economic rate. The money they pay is their commitment to what you are teaching them.'

After about 15 minutes of consultation, Elizabeth asked me to lie down on the table with my knees bent, and with my head resting on a pile of two or three books. The height of this pile depends on your height, and on how rounded the spine might have become. The point about the books is that they enable you to lie with a perfectly flat spine on the table.

Then when I was in position, she put her hands under my head and on my arms and legs in turn. As she did this, she asked me to 'give her the weight'. Here comes the first difficulty for many people. Instead of allowing her to take the weight of their head and limbs, they will try to help her. This is wrong. She wants people to go 'deadweight', so that she can search out the connections, and discover where the imbalances are.

The more tense and nervous people are, the less able they are to give Elizabeth their weight. They are, in some deep sense, afraid of 'surrendering' up to somebody who at this stage, is still a stranger. For extremely nervous and anxious people, just learning to let the teacher take their weight can take several lessons.

After that, Elizabeth moved round my body, touching muscles here and there. When she does this, it is hard to sense anything happening at all. There is no pain, no discomfort, no difficulty. I was just lying there, passively, while she touched particular muscles. Of course, this might hurt for people who have very bad muscular strain at a certain point but, even here, pain is unlikely.

The Technique does not involve jerking wrongly-placed joints back into position. It is not even like massage. What Elizabeth is doing at this stage is finding out how your muscles are positioned, what you have been doing to your spine, and where the problem areas are.

Most people do not realise that knees and ankles are actually connected to the spine, and cannot see why, when they have come with excruciating backache, Elizabeth spends so much time on their knee joints.

As she tests the muscles, she asks pupils to think of their spinal cords going right from their tailbone to the top of the neck and imagine it lengthening. She also asks them to let their neck muscles soften and release. All this takes about 20 minutes.

She then asked me to get off the table by rolling on to one side, then gradually lowering the legs on to the floor. This is achieved by putting the right arm over, and then following this through with the whole body.

I was then asked to stand with my back against the back of a chair. For a lot of people, this is quite difficult. Many people find it fairly easy to open out and release when they are lying down, but that this is quite a different matter when they are standing up. The reason for this is gravity. The teacher will ask the pupil to make the same releasing movement when standing as when lying down. This takes practice as, at first, many people do not understand what is meant by the term 'releasing'.

Next, Elizabeth put a cushion into the chair and eased me back into it, in the Alexander way. Here, you don't do anything, but let the teacher 'sit' you. This allows the teacher to observe what the relationship of the head to the spine is, and how far this is out of alignment. She chose this movement because I have some back problems. Again, most people find

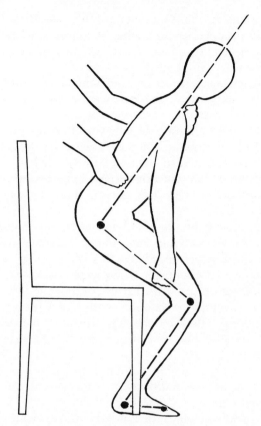

Working with the movements of sitting and standing

it difficult at first to sit in the correct Alexander way.

This first consultation takes about an hour, and forms the broad pattern of future lessons. In common with most modern Alexander teachers, Elizabeth Atkinson likes her pupils to have three or four lessons very close together, so that they get a good idea of what is happening. Otherwise, if there is too long a gap, they will forget what happens between one lesson and the next.

Further lessons – and homework

The 'homework' that Elizabeth sets her pupils is to lie down every evening in the Alexander position, perfectly still, and with head propped up on books, for about 15 minutes. They are also asked to practise sitting and standing in the Alexander way (see pages 24, 27 and 77).

During lessons, pupils will often not be aware that anything at all has happened. The realisation that muscles have actually been worked in very different ways usually comes the next day, when all sorts of aches and pains might set in. Although the method appears to be very gentle, people very often feel tired afterwards, and as if they have been exercising for a long time. The sensation that I experienced was as if I had gone for a very long swim. The feeling was not unpleasant, but achey.

When pupils come for their second lesson, Elizabeth will usually ask how the lying-down went, and what sensations, if any, the pupil experienced. At this stage, most people will completely forget about practising lying down – it has not yet become enough of a habit. Elizabeth will then spend a few minutes explaining the essential nature of this exercise.

'The more you do this,' she says, 'the more you get to know yourself. Ideally, you should get into the Alexander lying-down position every time you feel yourself under undue pressure. This has the effect of taking you out of your normal environment for a significant amount of time, and releases pent-up tension.'

Many people will find the lying-down surprisingly difficult because it is a discipline, and takes practice to achieve. It is quite hard to lie in one position without moving for 15 to 20 minutes. Physically, we are not used to it, but apart from that, as you lie you keep remembering things you must do, and the urge is to get up and do them, or to make a list of jobs. You have to resist these impulses, but it does not come naturally, at first. It is also, Elizabeth explains, quite taxing physically to lie down without moving for any length of time. Our bodies have become used to being in perpetual motion, at least when we are awake, and in some cases, simply *cannot* rest.

By the second lesson, the teacher will have gained valuable insights into the pupil's bodily strengths and weaknesses, and will have ascertained how free or 'locked' the head and neck have become. The second lesson usually concentrates more on enabling the head and neck to be free. Elizabeth Atkinson checks the joints, then comes back to the head and spine. 'It's like checking the powerhouse, the control room. Unless the relationship of head and neck can change for the better, there can be no permanent improvement.'

Patients who come for relief from a bad leg may be surprised to find that the teacher concentrates far more on their head and neck. But, the reason for the pain in the leg in the first place, is wrong 'primary control'. Whatever happens in the head, is reflected instantly to other organs, and all limbs.

Future lessons all follow basically the same pattern – a lengthy period of lying down, then practice in sitting and standing. They usually last for 45 minutes, as there are no further verbal consultations. As time goes on, more practices may be introduced. These may include crawling, squatting, and the famous 'expiration on a whispered ah'.

Unique to Alexander lessons, this is a procedure worked out by the founder to teach people the relationship between tightening the jaw and a narrowed rib cage. Unless you have flexible breathing, you can't hope for a flexible voice. The idea of breathing out on a whispered 'ah' is not to try and make a wonderful sound, but to allow the jaw to be freed and the ribcage to expand. All this happens naturally when the 'ah' comes out.

When you tighten everything, a tight sound emerges. Most people are simply not used to letting a sound come out as a result of thinking consciously. This practice also allows the back to be opened and widened.

Elizabeth explains: 'When you ask people to open and widen their backs, most haven't a clue what you mean. But if they do the whispered "ah", it happens naturally.' The exercise was developed to allow people to use their vocal cords without stress and strain. The process prevents sniffing and sucking in air. It does not allow undue depression of the larynx, muscles and vocal organs.

The whispered 'ah' can be practised by anybody, at any time. You place the tip of the tongue very lightly between the lower teeth and the rest of the tongue near the bottom of the mouth. As you do this, try to think of something amusing, or inconsequential, which makes you smile. If this is difficult, then try to imagine something lighthearted, which gives pleasure. As you imagine, open the jaw to let the sound 'ah' come out, not voiced, but whispered. As you do this, the chin should not jut out, but the mouth should drop forward and out. Repeat this three or four times.

As you make the whispered sound, you will notice that the ribs widen out. Do not overdo this practice, though, as it can cause hyperventilation.

Why practice is necessary

There may be more voice exercises in future lessons. The teacher may ask the pupil to make a series of sounds, to see whether too much effort is being put into speaking or singing. The teacher will also be watching to see if pupils pull their heads back as they speak. The whole idea is to make everyday movement effortless.

The idea of the lying-down exercise with knees bent is to encourage the back to open out. Unless the knees are bent, the back arches and tightens, and the lying down achieves very little. You will also be taught to give yourself specific instructions every time you change your movement. These instructions are: head forward and out, forward and up.

The sitting-down practice is to enable people to use their heels as weight-bearers, letting the knees go easy, and then easing back into the chair with the tailbone going first. You are taught to think of your spine as being all of a piece, and connecting up.

Future Alexander lessons may also include performing a Muslim-type prayer position. This gives people a very strong sense of what is happening to their backs. The teacher may ask the pupil to walk, and observe what is happening to their bodies as they do so. Very many people, without realising it, roll from side to side, and overwork the hips. A lot of people experience extreme discomfort when they walk for any length of time, but don't know why.

A favourite Alexander exercise is the 'monkey' position. The idea of this is to illustrate the anti-gravity principle, which is what the Technique is all about. Basically, the 'mon-

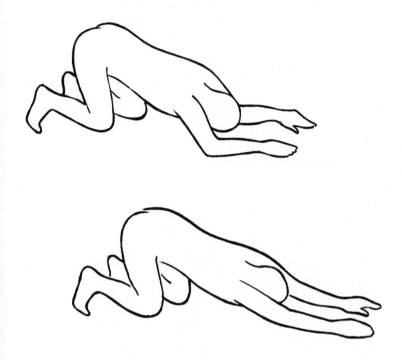

Muslim-type prayer position

key' is a stretch which lets the hips bend, and the pelvis straighten itself.

How many lessons?

Most Alexander teachers liken the lessons to fine-tuning an engine. After a few sessions, most pupils begin to see for themselves the connections between the spine and the muscles, the head and the neck, and start to 'feel the difference' when sitting, standing and lying down the Alexander way. The Technique takes quite a long time to establish itself in a person's mind and body and the number of lessons a particular pupil needs will largely depend on the problem they bring with them.

81

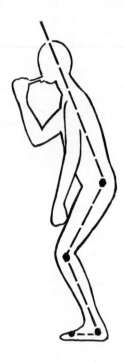

*Doing an everyday task
using the 'monkey position'*

Most people, said Elizabeth Atkinson, do not consider coming for lessons until they have had a major health crisis in their lives. Some people may be motivated by curiosity, but the great majority of pupils are people who simply cannot do their jobs any more, as their health problems have got so bad.

Most lessons are conducted on a one-to-one basis, as every person will have a different problem, and have developed a different use of the body. It is possible, though, to attend an introductory group course just to see what the lessons are like in advance, before committing oneself.

The immediate benefits of Alexander lessons is that tiredness at the end of the day can be overcome. Those who conscientiously do the lying-down after work will find renewed energy for the evening. The practice of giving yourself orders before changing position also works wonders. Nobody else need know that you are doing it. This ordering, says Wilfred Barlow, may be regarded as a 'pre-activity', something we tell ourselves before embarking on any action. Unless we remember to give ourselves these definite orders, we will be in danger of slipping back into the old, bad habits.

Becoming a qualified teacher

A question many people ask is: how will I know that my Alexander teacher is properly qualified? Can anybody set up as an Alexander teacher without going through a recognised course of training?

In the early days, it is possible that many people did set themselves up as Alexander teachers, without being properly trained. There was, and still is nothing to stop anybody setting up in practice, whether or not they have had proper training. But now, thanks to the formation of the Society of Teachers of the Alexander Technique, all teachers should be properly trained. The training is quite long and arduous, and only suitable people are accepted. Very often, trainees already have some other qualification in a related field, such as speech and drama or physical education, and have become interested in the technique en route. Very often, teachers are ex-pupils who benefited so greatly from their own lessons that they want to pass the teachings on.

Nobody can be accepted for training unless they have had Alexander lessons themselves, as a pupil, for at least a year. This ensures they will already have a very strong idea of what the Technique is all about. Many of the best teachers are people who encountered enormous problems of their own, and found that Alexander training was the only thing that helped.

The instructors at training courses are all Alexander teachers of many years' standing, and all courses must be approved by the Society. Courses are not usually residential, but full-time for three years. Most courses are small, consisting of no more than nine trainees.

The Society has checking procedures to ensure that all courses are properly run, and in the right Alexander tradition. There is now very strict quality control.

The three-year course covers 1600 hours of teaching. Each working week consists of a minimum of 15 workings hours, *not* crammed into evenings and weekends. It must take place in 'prime time', when the students are fit and alert.

The training course includes extensive instruction in anatomy and physiology. This is important, as nowadays many doctors refer patients to Alexander teachers, and the teachers often work with seriously ill people.

There are no exams, but pupils are given continuous assessment over the three years. At the end of the course, they can set up in practice as qualified teachers.

Anybody who is interested in booking up Alexander lessons can easily check whether the teacher is properly qualified, by asking if he or she is a member of the Society. If the teacher answers 'yes', but you still have doubts, you can contact the Society, which has a list of every teacher in the country.

Importance of rapport

In Alexander lessons, it is very important indeed for there to be a strong rapport between teacher and pupil. If you just don't 'click' with each other, it may be better to find another teacher, because you have to trust and co-operate with the teacher absolutely, and have confidence in his or her ability to help you. Sometimes, for no reason that can be easily explained, this essential rapport may not exist. You may find yourself resenting what the teacher tells you to do, for instance. If this is the case, it would be better not to continue. The very last thing that is needed is to experience added stress and strain, as the whole point of Alexander lessons is to *remove* undue tension.

Some pupils feel happier with a teacher of the opposite sex, whereas others are more at ease with an instructor of the same sex. As a lot of touch is involved, this needs careful thought beforehand. To gain maximum benefit from the lessons, you should positively enjoy and look forward to them. They are not, and are not intended to be, on a par with visiting the dentist or going into hospital, so there should be no feelings of fear, anxiety or tension.

The enjoyment which is felt when teacher and pupil are in perfect accord, is a very important part of Alexander therapy. Pupils should, however, be prepared for the possibility of some trauma. This does not happen with everybody, but those who are very ill or extremely tense may find that release of their problems causes unexpected, strong reactions.

Fiona Ross, the asthma sufferer first mentioned in Chapter 3, said 'After the lessons, I often walked home feeling physically on air, but inside, somewhat shaken. The lessons made me rethink my whole life, and ask myself what I was doing.'

Helen Dasquez, who says she will never stop having lessons as long as she lives, commented: 'They are the only thing in my life that has ever done any good, medically speaking. The money I spend on my weekly lesson has proved a wonderful investment. I have now, through the lessons, learned to take the many pressures off myself, and have time for myself. For me, they have now become a way of life.'

For Andrea Midlin, the lessons were a godsend when she had to look after her husband following a stroke. She said: 'I don't know how I would have managed without the lessons, as I had to lift my husband all the time. The main thing I learned is that a knowledge of the Technique completely alters the way you look at your situation. There is always a two-way traffic between mind and body, and the lessons help you to appreciate this.

'What the Alexander course did for me was to alter and recharge the batteries. I found that when you alter the 'means whereby' you do something, you can do everyday tasks with a better attitude, even down to the washing up. And all this has its important feedback to the mind.'

Andrea added that the Alexander Technique was not something you could just learn for a year, and then forget about. 'You have to include it in your everyday life, for the rest of your life. It is a new way of using your body consciously, and you need to keep working at it for ever. I was looking for something which would help me cope with my everyday life, and found Alexander lessons to be absolutely the answer.'

The next chapter looks at ways of incorporating Alexander wisdom into everyday life.

6

Putting it into practice

Although the Alexander Technique is not primarily a self-help therapy, it is possible to bring the basic principles into everyday use, without having lessons.

The three most important Alexander principles establish primary control. They are:

- Let the neck be free. Never increase muscle tension in the neck.

- Let the head go forward and up, never back and down to sit on and crush the spine.

- Let the torso lengthen and widen out. Do not shorten the back by arching the spine.

Sitting down

When sitting down, let your tailbone (coccyx) guide you, rather than plonking yourself on to a chair using your knees as the main joints. If you push your bottom out slightly, then lower yourself gradually on to the chair with the spine, head and neck naturally following, you will decrease the tension at the vulnerable joints. This way of sitting down must become a habit – and soon you really will notice the difference and wonder how ever you could have sat down in any other way. Make sure you do not ever cross your knees when sitting – you will never see an Alexander teacher doing this. For many of us, this has become a reflex, unconscious action, but in time will lead to bodily asymmetry.

In order to retain symmetry, you should ideally have your knees turned slightly outwards. Women have been taught that this posture is inelegant and it comes much easier to men. The correct Alexander way of being seated is much easier to achieve when wearing trousers or long skirts.

When getting up out of a chair, let your head go first and the rest of the body follow, rather than getting up with your knees, as most people do. Observe how people get up from a chair, and you will soon notice that most of them put a lot of unnecessary strain on their knees. The fluid, natural movement recommended by Alexander teachers actually makes standing up easier and leaves you far less tired at the end of the day. It is especially valuable for people whose jobs involve a lot of sitting and standing throughout the day.

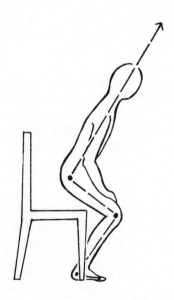

Getting up from a chair whilst letting the head lead minimises the downward pulls in the body

Lying down

This is an excellent Alexander procedure which anybody can practise at the end of the day. Ideally, it should be maintained for about 20 minutes. Those who have not attempted to lie perfectly still for such a long time will have no idea how difficult it can be. It is particularly valuable for hurry-hurry Type A people, who never give themselves enough time to do anything, and who are always impatient.

Lie on the floor, not on a bed, as this is too soft. Now place two or three books underneath your head – until your spine can go flat along the floor, and there is no arch at all. Have your arms at your side, and knees bent. Now just lie like that, breathing naturally, for at least 15 minutes; longer if you can. You will be amazed at how rested you become, and how much more energetic you feel when you get up again.

This procedure also teaches you about any imbalances in your body. Stiffnesses you were not aware of become obvious, and you will learn a lot about your own body and joints. This practice also enables the body to regain some of the symmetry it may have lost during the day, through bad usage, badly-designed chairs and car seats.

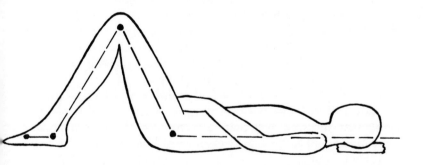

Lying on the floor with the head supported by an appropriate number of books helps the body to regain its natural alignment

The lying-down procedure also enforces relaxation, promotes proper breathing and gives a break from your usual routine. If you can, do this every single day, and get into the habit of lying down – possibly instead of having a gin and tonic when you get home from work in the evenings. Many business people have found it extremely useful when travelling and staying in strange hotels. It imparts new energy, and gives the strength to cope with a hectic evening programme even after a frantically busy day.

Understanding bodily faults

Since the way you now walk, stand and sit probably feels completely natural and normal to you, how do you know whether or not you are out of alignment? Wilfred Barlow has devised a simple test to enable people to ascertain this for themselves (see illustration opposite).

Stand with your back to a wall, with your heels about two inches (5 cm) from the wall, and feet about 18 inches (46 cm) apart. At this stage, do not let any part of your body actually touch the wall.

Now gradually press your body back to the wall, keeping your toes on the ground. If you are in complete alignment, your shoulder-blades and buttocks should touch the wall at the same time. If you are 'one-sided' you will notice that one side of your body touches the wall before the other side. If you hold your pelvis too far forward, your shoulders will touch the wall before your buttocks.

If this is the case, now bring your buttocks to touch the wall. You may be aware of a big gap between the lower back and the wall. Make this gap disappear by bending both knees forward, still keeping heels on the ground.

Dr Barlow says that anybody who is in a badly misused state will find this position tiring very quickly. But practice against the wall will help the stomach to lift and appear slimmer and tauter. This exercise will also encourage body realignment.

Chairs and seating

Bad postural and breathing habits develop and grow largely

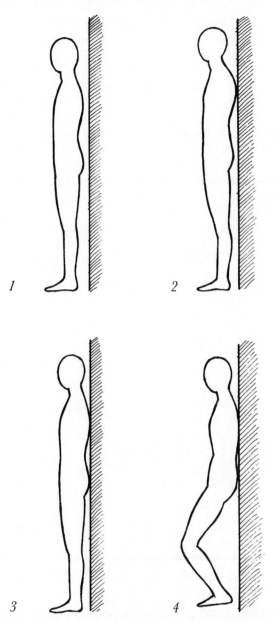

*This sequence done against a wall helps the individual
to apply his/her skills of inhibition and direction*

unconsciously. But of course, they are encouraged by sitting in the wrong kind of chairs. Few seats are designed on strict Alexander principles.

The 'Balans' type of chairs are perfect for spine realignment. Although some people find them hard to get used to, they are very good for those who have to sit at type-writers or VDUs all day, as they hold the spine erect, but not in an unnatural military-type position which encourages arching of the spine. Balans-type chairs are designed to trans-fer weight away from pelvic bones – another area which can easily become rigid and 'locked' over the years. They can also help people to avoid lower back pain, the main curse of today's sedentary worker.

Whatever type of chair you have, it is worth remembering, whenever you can during the day, to have your feet higher than your pelvis. Do this by putting your feet on a pile of tele-

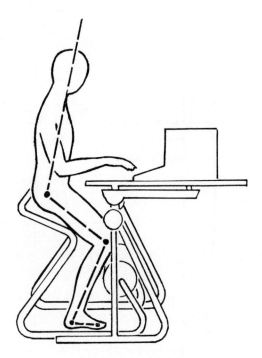

A 'Balans' type of chair

phone directories, on a stool, or perhaps a low table. It is not necessary to sit like this all day long, but the position helps to ease the pelvis and the spine, and so prevent backache. Pressure is relieved for those all-important minutes. Whatever you can do to break a bad habit of sitting or standing, said Alexander, also breaks a link in the chain which ties you to that habit.

Bear in mind that chairs do not exist in nature, and that they contort our bodies into unnatural positions, however good they may be. For this reason, it is a good idea to practise squatting as much as possible. Whenever you do not absolutely have to sit, squat instead. Those who have not squatted for many years may find this position difficult at first. But it is an excellent way of regaining body symmetry.

Posture

All the things we do in our everyday lives, such as driving cars, typing, ironing, gardening, picking up small children, housework, can cause or contribute to bad posture and thus to back and spinal problems. Few people ever stop to consider their posture, or what they might be doing to their bodies when they are rushing around doing all the jobs which have to be done each day. Driving is a prime example of how easily one can fall into bad habits. Nowadays, many people spend many hours each day in their cars and, with the advent of car telephones, this tendency is increasing.

Driving without pain

Most people who drive for a living, or whose job entails a lot of driving, sooner or later complain of bad backache. In fact, unless conscious attention is paid to posture, chronic pain will eventually accompany every journey. You have to make an effort to relax head and shoulder muscles, not to allow shoulders to hunch up with tension and not to lock the head back on to the neck. If you feel tense while driving, you can shrug your shoulders when waiting at traffic lights to release tension. Rolling the head from side to side also helps.

Humans are not designed by nature to spend hours sitting

at the wheel of a car, and it is all too easy to hunch over the wheel. When choosing a car, it is important therefore to choose a seat which gives firm, curved support to your back. A soft seat that you sink into is asking for back trouble. Ideally, the back of the seat should come up right to the top of your head, rather than end in the region of your shoulder blades. If your car does not have one of these, consider adding a neck support.

Correct lifting and gardening

There are right and wrong ways to lift things. All those whose job involves a lot of lifting should make sure they *never* bend over the child or the elderly bedridden person, or the item of furniture. That is just asking for back and joint problems. Keen gardeners should make sure they squat or kneel when weeding, planting and hoeing – and never bend their backs over their task. Those who have difficulty in getting into a kneeling position can now buy kneelers at garden centres: they are definitely worth having. When cutting lawns or hedges, do not do too much at one time, and if you have back pain avoid reaching above head height.

Above all, always get down to the task rather than bending over it. Handling heavy loads places great strain on the back, but as with everything else, there is a right way to do it. First of all, think about the 'means whereby' – rather than just getting the load from one place to another.

Many people, says Christopher Hayne in *Total Back Care*, have an objection to putting loads and crates next to their body. In fact, loads should be held as close to the body as possible. This is why people wear protective clothing in industry. It is also important to place your feet properly; they should be kept as far apart as your hips, with one foot slightly in front of the other so that you have a stable base. Try to keep the load between the base thus created by your feet.

Always avoid bending the spine when getting hold of a load. The spine should also remain straight and not twisted to one side or the other. Get down to the load with hips and knees. Do not grasp the load with fingertips, but with the whole hand, keeping the elbows tucked to the side of your body. This avoids stress on shoulders and neck muscles. Never attempt to pick up a load which is too heavy for you.

Observing reactions

People often imagine that they have no control over their own reactions to stimuli, whether pleasant or unpleasant. This is complete nonsense. If we so wish, we can train ourselves in our responses. Perhaps the best way to practise the Alexander Technique, and to minimise bodily imbalances, is not to over-react in any way. As reactions, like anything else, can become habitual, learning to respond in different ways can take practice and discipline.

But this does not mean it cannot be achieved. Next time something makes you angry, stop to consider whether your anger is really necessary, and whether it can achieve positive results. Very many people become angry when traffic lights turn red, when trains are late, or when people do not turn up for appointments. Whenever you feel angry, ask yourself: will my anger, however great, make any difference to this problem? If the answer is no, then start training yourself to respond calmly. All the anger in the world will not make a train turn up, or reduce a traffic jam.

Impatience, frustration and worry are basically acquired habits – and therefore they can be unlearned. Always ask yourself what positive results the frustration or worry will achieve. Worry, people have to learn, is an entirely useless emotion which serves no purpose. All worry does is to compound fear, anxiety and tension. Next time you watch a soap opera make a note of how often the characters 'worry' about each other. We interpret worry as caring about others – in fact, these two emotions have no connection! If you worry, you simply spread negativity without positive achievement. If you care, this means you have the best interests of the other person at heart, and need to remain in such a state to be able to think clearly about what they might need. Worry stops us from thinking clearly, and acting clearly.

Anxiety and fear are also largely learned responses. Of course, a certain amount of anxiety and fear act as protective mechanisms, but most of us go around with a far greater burden of anxiety and fear than is justified by the occasion. Correct Alexander-type breathing – deep and regular – does a lot to reduce fear. So does asking yourself: what is the worst that can happen? Will my anxiety have any positive benefits, either to me or anybody else? Usually, the answer will be no.

It is not easy to get rid of the kind of fear which has become habitual. But such fear always manifests itself in bodily postures. Learning to stand up straight, practising the Alexander lying down, and sitting properly, will all help to flood fear out of the system, and out of the mind.

American psychologist Susan Jeffers, author of *Feel the Fear and Do it Anyway*, says that the way to make groundless fears vanish is to do the thing you fear. If you fear public speaking, for example, force yourself to do it, on however small a scale. This will give you a sense of achievement and self-esteem which is vital for optimum health. Going around with an inbuilt fear destroys posture, body harmony and balance – and literally turns you into a nervous wreck. As we now know from our study of the Alexander Technique, you can never separate body and mind, but must enable the two to work well together.

Michael Gelb, author of *Body Learning*, says that most of us experience an almost habitual feeling of being on edge. This, he says, is a common over-reaction to the environment. His advice is to pause briefly when you hear the doorbell or telephone ring, instead of jumping up to answer them. This creates a calmness which will not be present if you rush to answer a ring.

Whenever we create extra calmness in our lives, this immediately transfers itself to bodily organs, muscles and joints. Also, whatever we do to minimise muscular overuse, will convey itself in extra calmness to the mind.

It is true that the Alexander Technique cannot be fully appreciated without expert lessons, but this doesn't mean there is nothing we can do to help ourselves. The fundamental principles described here hold good for everyday life, and will enable much distress to be dissipated.

Perhaps the most valuable lesson that can be learned from an understanding of Alexander therapy is that the condition of our minds and bodies is very much in our control. To a very great extent, we can choose good posture, correct body use and positive thinking – or we can choose to be misshapen, victims of ill-health and with a mind chock-full of negative, useless thoughts.

While nobody should underestimate the power of habit – and how much perseverance it can take to alter the ways of a lifetime – all those who have taken Alexander lessons and embraced the doctrines are in no doubt that it is eminently worth the effort.

Further reading

An A–Z of Alternative Medicine by B. Hafen and K. Frandsen. Sheldon Press, 1984.

Body Learning: An Introduction to the Alexander Technique, by Michael Gelb. Aurum Press, 1981.

Ends and Means, by Aldous Huxley. Chatto and Windus, 1940.

Eyeless in Gaza, by Aldous Huxley. Grafton, 1986. Contains a fictional portrait of F.M. Alexander and explains his fundamental teachings.

Feel the Fear and Do it Anyway, by Susan Jeffers. Century, 1988.

The Alexander Principle, by Wilfred Barlow. Arrow, 1984.

The Alexander Technique: Essential Writings of F.M. Alexander, edited by Edward Maisel. Thames and Hudson, 1974. Essential reading for serious students of the Technique, is now out of print, but can be obtained from libraries.

The Alpha Plan, by David Lewis. Methuen, 1986.

The Use of the Self, by F.M. Alexander. Dutton, New York, 1932. Reprinted by Methuen, 1987.

Total Back Care, by Christopher R. Hayne. Dent, 1987.

More information on Alexander courses can be obtained from: **The Society of Teachers of the Alexander Technique, 10 London House, 266 Fulham Road, London SW10 9EL.** Tel: 01–351 0828.

Index